About this book

Beloved Old Age – and What to Do About It is one of the variant titles that Margery Allingham gave to the book she usually called *The Relay*. Margery, who was born in 1904, was a crime novelist, famous for her Albert Campion detective series. From 1936 she and her husband, Pip Youngman Carter, lived in the village of Tolleshunt D'Arcy in Essex where her younger sister Joyce joined them in the mid-1950s. Joyce had bought a redundant blacksmith's forge across the square from Margery and Pip's home, D'Arcy House, and converted it into a cottage. In 1958, when the sisters took on responsibility for the end-of-life care for their mother, their aunt and an elderly cousin, Joyce's cottage was hastily developed into "dower house" accommodation.

When the period of care was over Margery wrote about the experience but the book was not published in her lifetime. She died in 1966, aged only 62. Her husband Pip and brother Phil did not long outlive her. Her sister Joyce remained in Tolleshunt D'Arcy until her own death in 2001. All of them were killed by cancer and none, apparently, had children.[1]

I was an Essex bookseller when I met Joyce in the mid-1980s. It was a friendship that had developed from a business approach when I applied for permission to re-publish her sister Margery's Second World War autobiography *The Oaken Heart.* Soon afterwards I began work on Margery's biog[...] friends and when she died I [...]eces of "unfinished business" th[...]f these

1 Pip had a son, Tom Carter, [...]

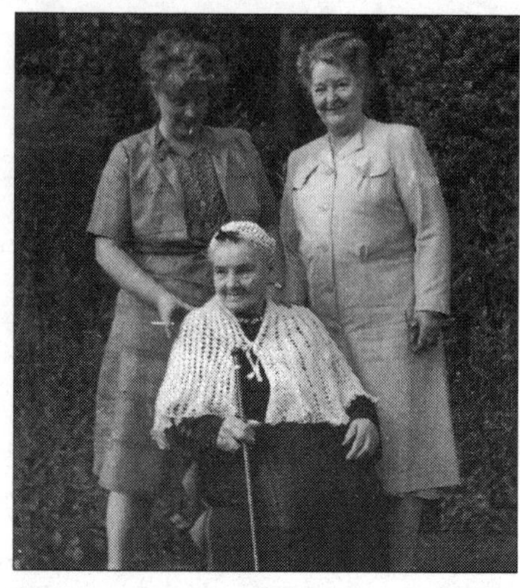

Three generations: Novelist Margery Allingham with her aunt and grandmother. She cared for them both in their final years.

was *The Relay*, a work which was particularly close to her heart.

By the time I first read *The Relay* in the 1980s it was already feeling dated. It had been written in a period which saw the beginnings of change in attitudes to the care of the elderly and the mentally ill. Peter Townsend's wonderful book *The Last Refuge*, published in 1962, had highlighted the plight of those thousands of men and women who were still accommodated in the Victorian Poor Law workhouses and public asylums that had been marked for closure in 1948 and there were other straws in the wind towards a greater kindliness in social policy through the humane, reforming 1960s. Now, fifty years later, the period atmosphere of *The Relay* provides an additional layer of interest as it encourages the reader to look back and to assess what has changed and what remains the same in society's attitudes to its oldest members.

Public arrangements are merely the context for Margery's book however. Its subject is the role of the family in the care of the elderly during the last years of their lives and that is the reason for my re-reading now. This has been a reading born out of necessity and I have interspersed my own current experience taking responsibility for my 92 year old mother, with Margery's chapters of advice – hence the change in title. *Beloved Old Age* is the record of a continuing process in which the idea of *The Relay* plays a central part. Margery was clear that hers was not "a book of personal reminiscence", though it springs from the events of her own life. I have very little other than my own (and my mother's) story to offer except that for the last eighteen months I have been involved, with my friend Nicci Gerrard, in John's Campaign.

John's Campaign begins from a very simple premise – that the carers and families of people with dementia should be welcome whenever the patient needs them, if that person is taken into hospital. Our analogy is with the 1960s campaign for parents to accompany their sick children in hospital and we hope that the attitudes of today's professionals will develop similarly towards an understanding of the need to work in partnership with those who are personally closest to the vulnerable and frail. Family carers are acknowledged now as they were not then but can still feel quite wrongly disempowered in their dealings with the caring institutions whether they be hospitals, residential homes or social work departments. *The Relay* challenges this. Individual caring is also a process that brings hard choices; guilt, anxiety, soul-searching, stress or exhaustion. *The Relay* insists that this can be worthwhile: that this stage of life can also bring shared laughter, happy memories and self-fulfilment and that seeing someone safely out of the world is as important as helping them into it.

I don't yet know whether Margery is right. My mother's story hasn't ended and the forthcoming anniversary of Margery's death and a recent birthday of my own reminds me that I have now reached the age at which she died. Nothing is certain in the ageing process when it is additionally complicated with illness. Cancer, rather than age, finished Margery's and her siblings' lives and was the scourge of her generation. Dementia is the preoccupation for many of my contemporaries and no doubt in another fifty years there will be something else. Human affection will still be around, and the desire to do the best we can for those closest to us, however imperfect our individual circumstances and abilities. The batons in life's Relay will need handing on again.

Julia Jones
May 2016

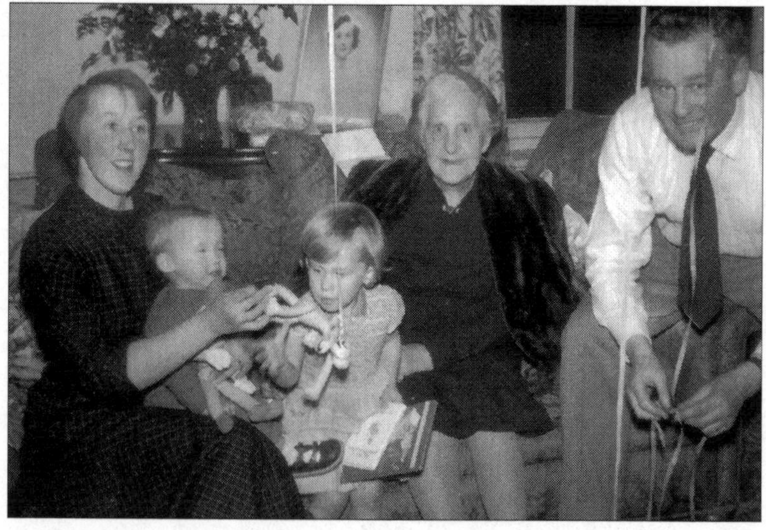

Three generations: June, Nicholas, Julia, Edith Maud & Jack Jones Christmas 1958

Beloved Old Age
And What To Do About It

Margery Allingham's
The Relay
Handed on to Julia Jones

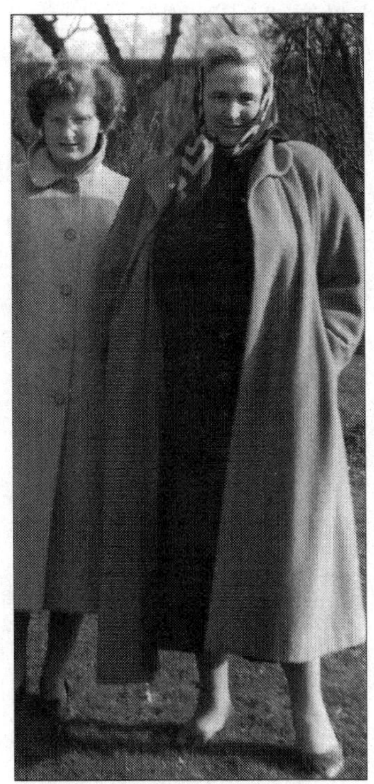

Joyce and Margery Allingham

This book is dedicated to my brothers, Nick and Ned

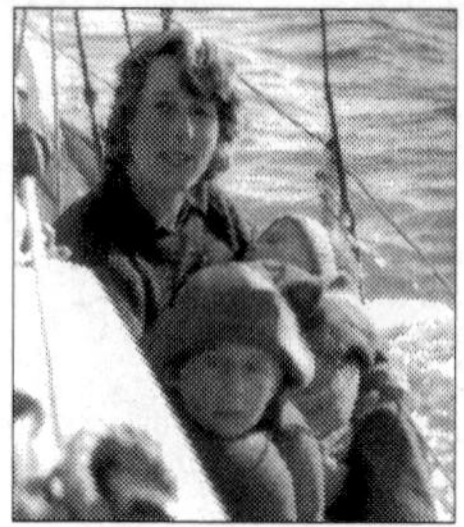

June, Nicholas and Edward Jones, Peter Duck, *1960*

First published in 2016 by Golden Duck (UK) Ltd.,
Sokens, Green Steet, Pleshey , nr Chelmsford, Essex CM3 1HT
www.golden-duck.co.uk

ISBN 9781899262298

Design by Megan Trudell

Ebook conversion by Matti Gardner

matti@grammaticus.co.uk

Printer and bound in the UK by 4egde Ltd, Hockley

Contents

Introduction: A family at its wits' end
Margery Allingham

A family at its wits' end settled the problem of caring for beloved but senile relatives (one with a stroke) by designing, building and running a self-contained bungalow, where every conceivable care could be given by one resident attendant and one visiting nurse, under the supervision of the family. Whilst this may not be the answer for all families, the lessons learnt are common to all and are set out for the guidance of those who still wish to take part in this very important stage of their own family history.

It was a private house solely used by the family (two sisters and a brother) to nurse in their last illnesses their mother and aunts, who each contributed only what they felt like paying towards the upkeep. As they were all senile their ideas of payment had little to do with the actual cost; the three heirs felt that the happiest way of ensuring their comfort was to lend them the extra money involved. Not only did the old people pay what they thought they would but the younger generation also contributed in unequal settled amounts according to their means. When the account ran out of money a small short loan was made by whoever happened to be in funds at the time and then was repaid when the account had money again.

Very careful records were kept by one of the daughters who was responsible for an analysis book with a separate banking account. In this particular family it was the daughter who lived and worked nearest and had the smallest income. She was the one to whom the resident Help first turned in the usual domestic emergencies that arose. She in her turn always had the head of the family available for the more important decisions and help. These details, of course, would need to be adapted to the family concerned.

When this particular household was no longer needed the younger generation found themselves enriched in knowledge not only about old age but about themselves. They were able to look back with happiness and humour to an important part in their own evolution and found it good.

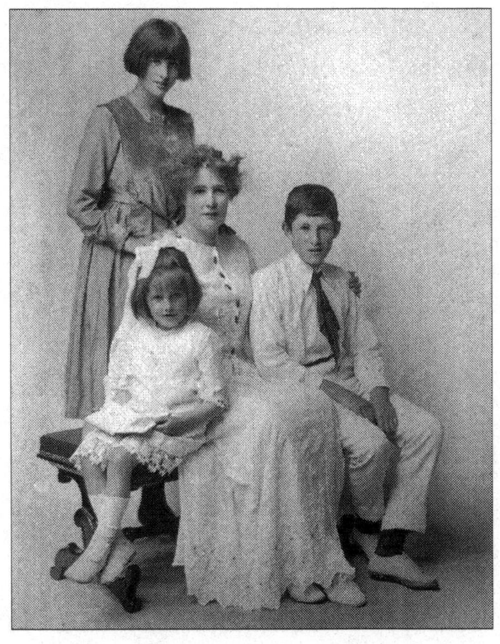

Em Allingham and her children c.1918

"And found it good"?
Julia Jones

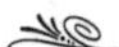

"They were able to look back with happiness and humour to an important part of their own evolution and found it good," says Margery. Did they? And can we? Or – if not we – can I? How?

I'm picking up *The Relay* at a time of need. My mother, in her 90s, is entering the later stages of Alzheimer's, my friend Nicci Gerrard and I have committed ourselves to a UK-wide campaign that is taking every scrap of energy that we have to give and then requiring more. I'm tired. I want to be with my partner Francis, with my children and my grandchildren, who are growing up much-loved but scarcely seen. Our boat, *Peter Duck*, will be seventy this summer. I want to go sailing. Above all, I yearn to write – elusive, unnecessary, adventure stories, not letters to Mum's doctor or Quality Measures for John's Campaign.

I know this won't last for ever. "It's only a phase" – as people say about toddlers and teenagers. But as toddlers and teenagers will understand, phases feel inescapable and eternal when you're "going through" them. Visibility is poor: the horizon closes in. It's easy to feel isolated, befuddled, depressed – even a little bit frantic. Remembrance Sunday in November regularly plummets my mother into a new low. It cannot be hidden, there are poppies on every lapel. She demands to attend the ceremony at the war memorial, to watch the march-past, to absorb the anguish of the last post and flinch at the exploding rocket that marks the end of the two minute silence. Then later she collapses, mentally, and I curse myself for giving in. I will never do so again.

Her distress is pitiable but also furious. It rocks us all. The weather worsens; the nights grow dark at teatime; the months ahead look grim. I hate the winters now.

Advice from friends flung me *The Relay* as a lifeline. I'd written a blogpost mentioning it: people sounded interested. I looked ahead, through the apparent impossibility of Christmas and the implacable approach of New Year, and realised that publication would be something to cling to; a small project that was purely mine, something manageable – with an end date. June 30th 2016, the fiftieth anniversary of Margery Allingham's death in 1966 sent out a signal like a racon.

Racons are radar beacons, fixed navigation marks that transmit their own distinctive beam. A racon on your screen is unmistakeable. It's a light in the navigational darkness. And, although anniversaries often appear to be manufactured events, I hoped that revisiting *The Relay* would offer me a way to think historically as well as personally, and so gain a longer view. *The Relay* was Margery's last completed book and has never previously been published. It mattered to her and she was glad to have written it, then she died months before it might have played some small part in a seminal campaign to improve the care of the old and the mentally ill. I've had *The Relay* in my mind for years, never certain what to do with it. Key ideas and individual phrases have glimmered like small flashpoints since my first reading in the 1980s. In that dark November, publication to mark the half century since Margery's death offered me something definite to steer for.

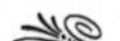

"If you want to make God laugh," says Nicci, "tell him your plans." I'd made the decision to publish *The Relay*: I wasn't certain how. Already the weeks were drifting by but this evening was free. I'd finished my tasks so I made my excuses and retired upstairs to think. How should I structure this book? Its pages were spread across the bed, my laptop was open, my pen in hand. I had the beginnings of an idea. My heart beat faster. The phone rang. I ignored it.

"Sorry," said Francis, "It's someone from Deben View."

Deben View is the extra care housing scheme where my mother has a flat. We have an understanding that the staff there will always ring (or help Mum to ring) if she's upset beyond their power to comfort. This means frightened, disorientated, enraged, paranoid, violent – or any combination of these. The carers who work in Deben View are truly good, kind people who understand that Mum's illness means that she can't always think or communicate clearly. They accept that her wilder moments are an expression of desperation, a scream for help, so when the situation is running out of control, they ring me. The arrangement is simple. I need to tell her I love her and help her calm down. She needs to recognise my voice, listen to my reassurance and come back to herself.

On this particular evening Francis and Georgeanna, my daughter, were in the room next to the telephone when they were startled by a furious screech from me: "Just go off and die then, you silly cow!" Mum, in her flat at Deben View, threw down the phone and came back, threw it down again and came back once more, shouting at me all the while as I shouted back at her that it was extremely rude to shout at people and *her* mother would have been ashamed of her and so was I – all at full shout. This appalling conversation did in fact end up with Mum calmer and me only moderately hysterical, but there was no more work to be done that evening. I stayed sitting on the floor, my back against the wall, my hand over my eyes, battered by emotion.

I often think of a young man who allowed himself to be quoted in a dementia support guide: “I loved my mum more than words can ever express but dementia could turn her and me into monsters that I did not recognise.”[2] I wish I could say that I didn’t recognise this monstrous aspect of myself but that wouldn’t be true. It wasn’t only that this phone call had shattered a moment that had seemed so breath-holdingly full of promise, it had reawakened the crosswinds of hurtfulness and quarrel throughout our lives. Among the many reasons that I find comfort in *The Relay* is that Margery and her mother, Em Allingham, never had a trouble-free relationship. Neither did her sister, Joyce.

Joyce was the front-line daughter most frequently called upon for help in “the usual domestic emergencies” over *The Relay* period. We were friends in her own old age and I cherish her memory. Joyce told me that she had lived most of her life learning to avoid her mother but, when Em could no longer survive alone, this lifelong antagonism became of secondary importance. There was intense wariness and worry at the prospect of care. There may have been rows (what Margery describes as a “thundering emotional upheaval”) but there wasn’t finally any doubt that Joyce and Margery would accept responsibility for their mother and their “own” old people. *The Relay* insists (and Joyce confirmed) that they were glad that they did so.

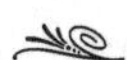

2 *A Road Less Rocky: Supporting Carers of People with Dementia* (Carers Trust 2013).

The day in the summer of 2010 when my mother's illness was diagnosed as Alzheimer's disease was a defining moment for us both. I had expected that the doctor would confirm vascular dementia – which for some unscientific and completely erroneous reason I was predisposed to find acceptable. This duly happened and I was beginning to stand up, collect our coats and take leave of the Memory Clinic when I realised that the doctor hadn't finished. Mum's MRI scan had also revealed extensive damage caused by Alzheimer's.

This information was almost impossible to take in. How could anyone have *both?* It wasn't *fair* (that cry of childhood). I remember very little more except the doctor's ruffled white blouse and lacy sleeves, the leaflet which she gave me advertising mobility aids and then the extraordinary instruction that it was somehow up to me to research a drug called Aricept and decide, together with the GP, whether or not Mum would be taking it. How could this be *my* responsibility? I had thought that prescribing medicine was what doctors did...

My youngest brother, Ned, and a friend were setting out on a brief holiday. They diverted as soon as they heard the bad news and called at Mum's flat to offer comfort. Ned was talking lovingly with Mum: his friend and I were making conversation. English wasn't her first language and I knew that she was doing her best in an awkward situation. I remember listening with appalled amazement as she told me that my mother was "going on a journey" and that I would be travelling "on the journey with her". My resentment was gigantic, completely disproportionate. I hope that I managed to stay speechless. Then she and Ned climbed into her converted camper van and continued on their way to the Welsh hills. Six years later it still doesn't quite calm me down to accept that she was right.

In addition to the racon there's another unmistakeable pattern of signals which one hopes not to see on a nautical radar screen. It's a stream of dots indicating the position of a SART, a Search and Rescue Transponder. This means there's a vessel in distress. It's a Mayday and wherever you thought you were heading at that time, the law of the sea demands that you turn towards the source of the distress and make all possible speed to offer assistance. When an emergency comes most families will do the same. But the crises of beloved old age may last for months or even years. This is a shipwreck in slow motion.

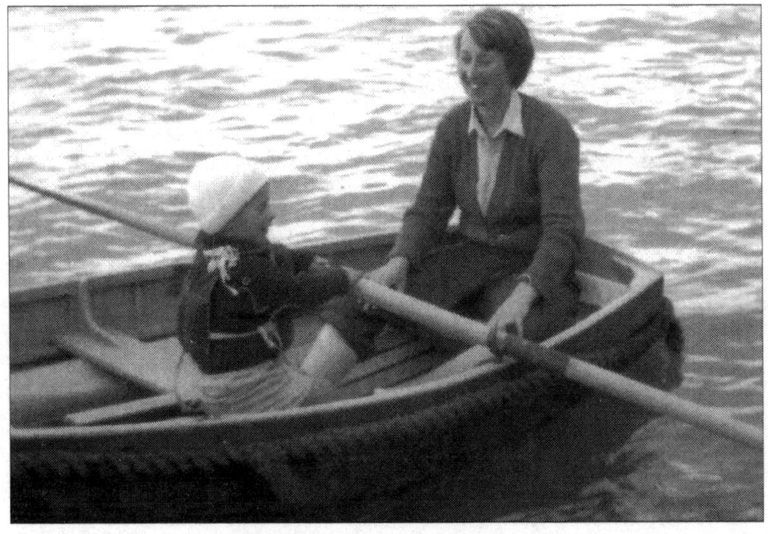

Julia and June Jones summer 1956

"The young crows don't feed the old crows!"
Margery Allingham

"The young crows don't feed the old crows!" My father, whom I loved very much, used to quote this to me as a child and it made me irritable and him depressed.[3] What good it did either of us I do not know, unless it serves to illustrate this piece and is probably the reason why I ever thought of writing it. The fact remains that whatever the popular cynicism of the period, men are not crows. All but the most afraid or the most inept do make some attempt to look after their old people, in some cases proceeding to lengths of self-sacrifice which are positively neurotic. It is a natural instinct in the human being who is not degenerate, and a very powerful one.

In doing so, many of the emotional hazards as well as the practical ones come fresh to the younger generation and often produce in the most conscientious a feeling of isolation. The existing literature tends to be technical, but the subject is like God and the drains: if you need to know about it, there is nothing you want to know about more or quicker. This does not pretend to be a treatise on geriatrics but its aim is to set on paper some practical aspects of a delicate and difficult adjustment to modern times and to list one or two methods of approaching it. These were discovered by trial and error in a period of transition and are set down for the instruction and convenience of those in similar

3 Margery's father was Herbert Allingham (1867-1936).

circumstances who see this personal problem drawing near.

I think perhaps I should first make it clear that in attempting this small book about old age and the family I have had the prudence to wait until I am able to speak with some authority. Now at sixty, my view of this subject must be approaching near an old person's own.[4] It was not always so. When my grandmother died at one hundred after living with me for the last ten years of her life, my brother and sister and I, who had full lives of our own, were then called upon to consider the care of our mother, her sister and her cousin, one after the other. We felt that the problem of the old people was one which must be approached with more than haphazard goodwill if we ourselves were to survive to become problems in our turn.

From an elderly point of view one does not have to consider the question of old age very long before it is clear that all one's life one has been taking part in some kind of relay race, and that the period of age is that portion of it in which one passes the baton to the next sprinter. For a while we must run together and during that time everything that is of value to the team passes from hand to hand. When the handover is taking place the whole family and those in-laws involved, and not necessarily those of one blood (although blood, I suspect, is more important than this particular period reckons), is in a state of emotional flux. Never is there such hypersensitivity between brothers and sisters as when father and mother are "going", although the process may take a decade or even two. It is a delicate time rather than a purely painful one, but like every other phase in life it can be a rewarding session or a terrible one, a thrill or a misery.

Receiving the baton is a tricky business just as is handing it over. The process is often bedevilled nowadays by an

4 Margery was born in 1904.

element of imagined guilt. There has been such a fashion for depreciating old ways of thinking that the whole idea of inheriting anything has become sullied. Yet if one does not look forward to one's inheritance one does not look forward to life. Inheritance is not merely something one has not earned. That idea has only become general since governments have found it necessary to take so much of the material part of it away. Nor is there anything narrow about the term. Inheritances vary. The only thing they have in common is that they are real, definite items one did not have before one inherited. The most important legacies in the long run usually turn out to be "unfinished business" and nothing material at all. Also, they are always a surprise.

If one does not only inherit goods, it is also true that one is seldom the only legatee. During the handover each person often appears to have several batons each of which are given separately. In one's time one inherits all sorts of things and one should be on hand at the right moments to take what is not a gift but a right and a responsibility. Some batons one recognises at once and knows when one has received them, whoever has given them. Some are important and some are just delightful things to have.

One cloudless day this summer I was listening to an old man who was talking of his life when he was a boy in Hertfordshire, helping his grandmother, who was a maker of bulrush baskets. As we stood in a garden, we saw a charm of goldfinches dancing over and over each other like a team of tumblers. They were splendid, their gold and crimson flickering on the other side of a hazel bush against the bright blue sky. He was telling me he had learnt from his grandmother that their country name was "King Harrys".

I was wondering what that old lecher, Henry the Eighth, had to do with such lovelies and whether he ate them, when it came to me that I saw something very like this pretty sight almost every day. On the boxes of typing paper which I use there is printed the arms of the Plantagenets: golden lions on scarlet, golden lilies on azure in quartering. So it was England's earlier King Harry, the conqueror of Crecy and not the Tudor monarch, whose shield and surtout flickered through the leaves five hundred years ago reminding the country folk of the other sight they knew which was so brave. This crest is a very pretty medallion and my friend, who is almost eighty, gave me a pearl to hang on it. He mentioned that the siskin, that little grey-green bird who sings and builds at the very tips of the fir trees, used to be called "The Ever Divine". That is nothing to throw away either.

That baton was for me. I took it and I pass it on here to any young runner who will carry it down the years. Frequently one is not aware that one has received a baton until the time comes when one needs it. They range from the instant recognition that the spots on a child are not erysipelas or the plague but a harmless family malady for which the cure is so-and-so, to the sudden realisation, perhaps long after the older person has gone, of who exactly one is, where one has come from, what one has been doing with one's life, why one has had it and, quite possibly, a pretty fair glimpse of the sort of future which is opening out before us when it is our own time to hand over.

In this country we have spent many generations building our complicated civilisation into a tremendous piece of mechanism. It seems absurd to turn it over to a new shift of technicians every thirty-five years, expecting each new team to rediscover the necessary skills for running it. Perhaps I may leave the subject by saying that I do not believe that the benefits are ever all on one side and that Auntie leaves a great deal more than her Gilts.[5] Some of her bequests are pieces of her own or Uncle's life work, necessary to her heirs for the structure, or the journey, or the piece of evolution that we are all undertaking whether we know it or not.

In common with all the great manoeuvres in life, the hand-over has a ritualistic inner pattern of its own. This can be ignored by those who prefer to, but for those who are anxious to live every part of life, to enjoy it and see what it is about, here is one way of achieving the goal without upsetting the contemporary home. First we must consider exactly what it is to which we are referring. According to Doctor Reginald Southey of Barts, writing nearly one hundred years ago, the period of advanced life is sixty to eighty-two and old age from eighty-two onwards. These figures seem remarkably good for people who had not the advantages of our improved medical knowledge and it would be surprising if any pundit today put them much higher.

The Victorian was speaking of the survivors, of course, but it may be that medicine and old age have not very much to do with one another. The one thing about age on which everybody agrees is that it sets in insidiously and sometimes early on. Perhaps it is at the instant when something emerges from the ovens of our experience completely and thoroughly done that the process begins. Physically the symptoms are so well known and so often discussed and tabulated that they hardly bear repeating, but usually this is observed from the outside. From the inside, getting old feels very like wearing out a favourite pair of shoes which slowly become uncomfortable and awkward

5 Gilts were a form of safe Government investment which many people used to provide a small regular income. In an earlier version Margery wrote Consols, which were the Victorian equivalent.

but never strange. One never changes. That first childhood's memory of oneself thinking something, however brash and bright, never turns into somebody else. After that first meeting it is always Me in Another Hat.

From the point of view of the younger members of the family who are waiting on them, elderly people seem to disappear into a hard shell of preoccupation with their own care and needs. Their world shrinks visibly until it reaches the size of that area round their chairs that can be reached with an arm or at least a stick. Sometimes one can rouse them and then they emerge with a flash of their old charm. It does not last, they sink back into a fastness where it becomes harder and harder to get near them. I wonder if this may not be an illusion of an optical kind. That which looks like a shell is really an absence; one moves slowly out to one side of the track and one looks across when summoned.

The first signs of age which most people observe in themselves are impaired sight and an impaired frontal memory. That is to say the failure in the memory for affairs which one experiences in youth when one is tired. If when sewing the scissors seem always to be missing, or if when writing the right word or train of thought is lost, one says cheerfully: "I *am* tired." When this happens in age one feels first exasperated and then perhaps frightened.

I can see already that the characteristic urgency of old age: "I must do what I have to do NOW!", "Let me tell you this NOW!", "You must give me my pen NOW!" may spring from nothing more mysterious than the failure of this kind of memory. Indeed, the more one examines the subject the more one sees that tiredness, with all its familiar signs, is the prime symptom and that as one behaved in one's youth and middle age when one was tired, so, the chances are, one will behave when one is old. Some of us protest and some of us retain angelic forbearance and control and most of us withdraw quietly and indicate that we do not want to play anymore.

This moving out on to the edge of the track is instinctive and we notice it instinctively. Some people, who perform the whole manoeuvre of the handover in the Relay beautifully and finish their sprint and go back to the pavilion amid general praise, never notice the operation any more than do some children who sail through puberty without a fear or a boil. The performance is natural and we prepare for it in that curious, complicated way in which nature goes about such things. Wonderful but unlikely and almost amateurish developments and aids appear as the need for them arises. This is true of every aspect of the story but I speak now of the mental and emotional one which most concerns the younger people involved.

This is no place to start talking about leaving the field or the importance of getting a fairly sound if rough idea of where one is going; although I think perhaps I should mention that, in my experience, the moment of truth is not when an old person realises that he is going to die one day, but the moment when he suddenly sees that this is not entirely true. The young sometimes make the mistake of thinking that the interest which one begins to take in a future existence, sometimes for the first time very late in life, is because one is loath to believe that living is over. This is not so. What has happened is more disconcerting. One has observed that it is not over at all. Having assumed, sometimes quite happily, that one is advancing on a blank wall, one has suddenly perceived that there is a door in it which shows distinct signs of opening. This can be a shocking discovery but the shock passes quickly, as if it were only the intellect which had ever opposed the idea. The rest of the body and personality appears to accept it as a natural discovery about itself.

What happens after that point is entirely a matter for the individual; all I would like to say here is that I believe that those intellectuals who are apt to say affably over the air, "Of course, I don't believe in a deity or survival after death" can have no idea to how many of us they are as acutely embarrassing as if they had prefaced their dissertations on Life and Art with the information that they belong to a sect who know for a fact that the earth is flat. The most surprising thing one learns as one grows older is that, whether one likes it or not, one has a faith and one puts it firmly in something, be it only a pill.

When one is preparing to go anywhere there is a hiatus in time, a moment when one must step off one path on to another, and one sees it coming, sometimes for a long while. If one is obstinate about making up one's mind one can put other people in some agonising dilemmas. I remember my own helpless dismay when a well-loved and thoroughly "good" but completely agnostic relative, who had always been an authority in my life, on desiring reassurance after her second stroke, suddenly commanded me to send for the police.[6]

Meanwhile, there are lesser items to think about which are also important. A thing we will all have to face, while we still care about it, is that we are going to get bored with the affairs which hitherto we have found fascinating. I know that a great many people who have not reached sight of that juncture are reluctant to believe it, but "The day I do not look at the stock market report I shall be dead" is in the same category of remarks as the "Everybody should be 'put down' at forty" of the twenty-year-olds. I had one old friend who could not bring

6 Evidence elsewhere suggests that this was Aunt Maud Hughes.

herself to believe that the time would come when she could not manage her own affairs. She carried the theory to the point of absurdity by retaining but delegating all the wearisome details more and more casually to anybody who happened to be about. She lived deep in the country and she got absolutely anyone who called at the door to write the letters of instruction to her solicitor for her. It seemed afterwards that every half-wit on earth had had a shot at it with the best will in the world. Her solicitor was either idle or old himself, her estate was minute and the easiest way for him was to act upon these staggering documents. A series of miracles alone saved her descendants their patrimony, which was not negligible when they got it, the estate being in land which rose in value.[7]

This withdrawal from affairs is a matter of degree. We do not become incapable of management in the clear-eyed way in which one becomes incapable of standing if one breaks both legs. Rather, we slowly grow to feel that business is not as rewarding as it was. If one is leaving a chair one does not kick it over and break it behind one. For that reason it is best to find two trustworthy people to take one's place while one can still be bothered to arrange it. There are people, who having left all this too late, make themselves miserable worrying over just this problem.

From my own present position with one foot in either camp, it seems to me that the only plans the old person can make for any sort of practical future are first to find his heir, next to find his solicitor to protect them both and then to decide if he is happier working or just sitting about. I do not think it matters which. What he is about to do is to ripen and become his own irrevocable self. I think most adult people

7 If the reference is to Cousin Grace the estate would be Pope's Hall, subject of Margery's 1955 novel *The Beckoning Lady*.

know this before they reach anything like old age. The old never want sudden death. If they insist that they are "ready" it merely means that they think the process must be complete, sometimes a little while before it is.

One of the very strange things about inheritance is that the main heir is not always apparent. One does not choose him, it seems; he "emerges". He is the person who assumes responsibility and is not necessarily the recipient of the material baton. Sometimes he is there from the beginning, the obvious person, but this is not always so.[8] The wisest of us, both old and young, let what is to happen happen, without fuss or heartburning.

Very often the most difficult thing for the heir to face is that he must not hold up his own sprint. Because the previous runner is fumbling with the main baton, they must not both sit down. Nor is he being any more filial or virtuous if he sacrifices the latter half of the race to the earlier one. For the time being he is in charge of the whole. Everybody knows all this, of course, but it is often very difficult to consider natural things simply in an artificial world.

Do not make the mistake of trying to save money by cutting out the solicitor. A good solicitor is the best substitute for one's own common-sense in any crisis which may arise. Honesty, intelligence and above all interest are what one is looking for in him. Let us not choose a man older than ourselves. Young solicitors often look after old people very well. After all, one is more likely to require hard work from them than abstruse legal advice. Above all one should avoid the amateur; someone has

8 Margery's papers show her making a conscious decision to direct *The Relay* at a male reader. She explained that she was attempting to give men confidence that they could cope with what they might otherwise regard as "women's business". Joyce later commented that she didn't see many men getting involved, "even in these emancipated times".

to be trusted and the legal profession tries to make a job of this and has some formidable machinery for enforcing trustworthiness in its members. It is worthwhile spending a lot of time and thought finding the right young man.[9]

There are some people who put their full trust in doctors, which is frankly dangerous. The new civil-servant medico is an over-worked man and the Doctor Camerons, with their omniscience and their passionate mercifulness, cannot now afford to be quite the fellows they were when they had all those long gig and brougham rides in which to think about the people they had seen.[10] Doctors, too, are notoriously some of the worst businessmen in the world, if also by far the most well-meaning. Also, they are the most used to having to take some sort of immediate action. That is not an ideal combination in an amateur adviser.

A good doctor is one of the most valuable people an old person can know but because of this we are liable to forget the one really curious thing about him. From the age of twenty-four or so, until he is almost too old to speak, he is the only person in the modern world whose lightest word is not only listened to by everyone he meets, but whose advice is taken and acted upon as if it were the instructions on one of his own bottles. While he sticks to his own subject he is reasonably infallible but if he strays from it: "At your age, what can you expect from the future?" or "In my opinion your son Henry is more trustworthy than your son George" – he can easily be as wrong as anybody else.

It is this business of finding those hands one can trust which usually causes most of the indecision and unhappiness so

9 Arrangements such as powers of attorney have changed but the advice to think ahead about whom one would choose to entrust with money matters or well-being arrangements remains good.

10 Reference is to the BBC TV series *Dr Finlay's Casebook* (1962-1971).

common at this time of life. The problem, too, is aggravated by modern conditions. Before the late nineteenth century, which was so determined to have "everything and heaven too" that it very nearly lost the lot, no adult expected to be able to put his trust in anything mortal and, I imagine, life and death were the easier for it. Even now, halfway through the greatest "operation clay foot" known to history, one still finds people who expect to be able to lean on something concrete and man-made.

For the old person the point of let-go is extremely difficult. Anyone who has ever given a power of attorney knows what a mental and emotional leap it entails. If one has never accepted a supreme authority it is now that one probably turns one's attention to the reliability of the family. If one is then beset by doubts about Mary being too like the Robinsons or George having a streak of Uncle Joe in him, it is as well to remember that the mug who trusts everybody has always appeared to fare better than the one who trusts no-one.

If one trusts everybody one at least puts the onus on them. They start thinking about trust anyhow, and their instinct, if they are pleasant, is to watch and protect one. If they are not pleasant they take advantage and rob one. As our entire civilisation is based on there being more social than a-social or anti-social people in existence we are more likely to be protected than cheated. If one trusts nobody, nobody cares what happens to one. Anyhow, the only person we can be absolutely certain is going to prove really untrustworthy in X years' time, as sure as eggs are eggs, is oneself.

If one's basic temperament does not alter with age except in intensity, its hard fruit does become more obvious as the obscuring graces drop away. The work done or not done on oneself over the years shows now and we declare our handiwork to those who are most like us; we show them our considered version of the pattern which they share with us.

There are all sorts of catches about this invaluable presentation. For instance, the effects of physical trouble on the mental and emotional condition have hardly begun to be understood. Medicine is only playing round the home slopes of this subject now, and because it is just becoming clear that much temperamental trouble is medical we have rather given up the older approaches to the subject.

The examples are endless: the woman who has a highly developed gay, proud, jealous, imaginative and generous disposition, (explosive enough as a mixture to have needed a firm hand all her life) can be transformed by quite a small amount of toxication into a fiend. A family of daughters can be driven almost insane by a condition of the thyroid gland in their mother, since every unreasonable symptom of hers appears to be a blown-up version of one of their own known and controlled temperamental weaknesses.[11] The mental symptoms of the toxic effects of constipation, of indigestion, of bronchitis, are none of them generally recognised by the family. The woman who takes regularly an old-fashioned bromide medicine to get to sleep, without realising what is happening to her, can easily pass for senile, and that not only with a lay audience. Before deciding that an old person is "impossible" it is as well to give one's mind to every aspect of his physical condition.

However, when all that can be done has been done and even when health is perfect, the temperament and the fruit of it remain. We become set not only in our ways but in ourselves. Our raw spirit has been put through clay and the refining process is almost over. Our conclusions have been drawn. It is

11 Both Margery and her mother suffered from poorly controlled thyroid conditions.

now that our heirs must look out for themselves because we do not always recognize immediately what has happened to us. When we see a younger version of our own mixture we see a pattern so like our own once was that we sometimes feel it is ours and we want to have another go. Or else we think we see it developing differently and decide in a panic that it is going wrong. We are missing, of course, the important fact that the life is not ours but his, and even if he wants help with the subject, which is unlikely, we cannot give it to him. All we can do is to show him ours for what it is worth.

Another unexpected and often misunderstood difficulty arises because we are so much ourselves. Our main machinery remains and when we are roused from our present preoccupations to deal with some factual situation which would be new to us at any age, we use the mechanisms we always did use, forgetting that our years have altered the picture. That can make us unreasonable and very hard to take. I am thinking for instance of the woman who has always secretly felt herself her daughter-in-law's rival. On finding herself suddenly in that younger woman's home she may begin to behave as if at last she has vanquished an enemy and has got what she had always set her heart on – sonny's house and sonny's love and sonny's children. In vain she may remember perfectly well that they are not for her. She may know she has other things to do and think about but very often, to her own dismay, she goes on behaving like a lunatic because she has no other mechanism with which to meet the powerful emotional situation.

Presumably one should have lived so intelligently that one's machinery is foolproof whatever happens but this is a tall order and the best of the lesser counsels in my experience is to learn to mind one's manners. It is an extraordinary fact that the very last thing one relinquishes are one's manners, if one has any. One encounters and hears examples of it time and again. I remember my grandmother, who had been bedridden for some years and was being turned over by myself and my sister at the end of a tired finish to a long, long life.[12] Suddenly she looked from one to the other of us and said brightly and distinctly: "I don't know who you are but I am sure I am very much obliged to you." Had we been disgruntled municipal workers or archangels we should have been just as gratified and touched as indeed we granddaughters were. So she was armed for any situation, including a world of new people.

Another valuable which seems to remain one's very own is one's skill in one's craft and every time we practise it we are as much in our prime as ever we were. The happiest old people I have ever met, in a lifetime of meeting a great many, are those who are still permitted to do something which they always did do superlatively well – making the giblet pie, planting the roundel of beans, crocheting the pattern, writing the sentence, playing the air.

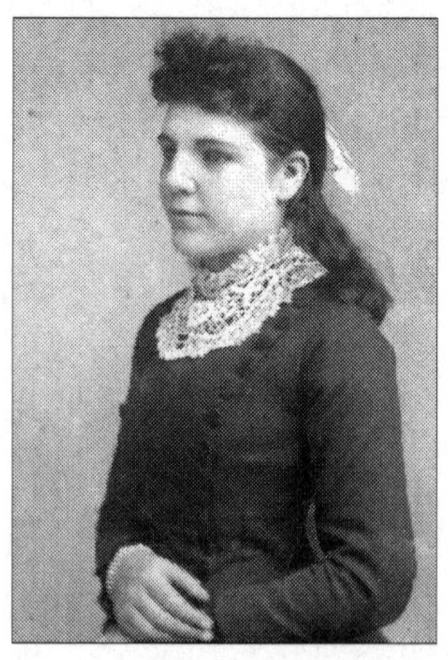

12 Margery and Joyce's grandmother was Emily Jane Hughes (1852-1952).

"Writing the sentence, playing the air"?
Julia Jones

Maud Hughes, Margery and Joyce's aunt and one of the three old ladies whose care at the end of their lives is the subject of *The Relay*, was not one of those happy elders who would settle contentedly to crochet a pattern or make a giblet pie.[13] She was a Fleet Street editor who had begun her career during the First World War working on the *Daily Sketch* and had then become co-editor of *Woman's Weekly*. After the war she had founded *The Picture Show*, Britain's first magazine for film fans. For almost forty single-minded years her magazine was her passion. She had no children, kept her marriage an open secret (so she was not debarred from working) and preferred the "business girl" to her "dull stay-at-home sister".[14] In 1958 she suffered a stroke after a showing of Cecil B de Mille's epic film *The Ten Commandments* and was forced to retire.

Without her magazine, Maud could not be happy and she didn't bother to pretend. A visiting colleague wrote to Margery; "We were sorry to find Miss Hughes so bleak because she really is in clover. Everything there is so beautifully bright and fresh. What more could one want? It scarcely seems possible for one to change so much. Do hope she will soon snap out of it."[15]

Margery knew enough to understand why Maud would not "snap out of it". "She wanted to be in her office and managing

13 Maud Hughes (1884-1961).

14 From a *Woman's Weekly* editorial, quoted in *Fifty Years in the Fiction Factory,* Julia Jones (Golden Duck 2012).

15 Letter to MA from Joy and Hulme Chadwick (1959).

her people and because she was not well enough to do that, she sulked." Sulked is a harsh word yet some very close families do describe each other's behaviour in terms that make an outsider blink – and which would be completely impermissible for any outsider to use. Margery is accepting her aunt's behaviour, not judging or trying to change her. One of the strongest themes of *The Relay* is the need to be near your family (or those closest to you) at the end of your life because they already know what you're like. There's no pretending required. It's safe for them to see your final self.

I modified the word "family" in order to make the obvious point that families may not necessarily share their DNA. Margery herself believed that the importance of "blood" might be underestimated but, fifty years later, we are increasingly aware of the variousness of family types and the extent to which families can be made, not born. The word "familiar" is a good one, describing those people with whom we are most comfortable, most naturally ourselves. Whatever network of relationships provides that fundamental acceptance to any particular individual, the message of *The Relay* is that Families Matter.

After DD-day (Dementia Diagnosis) how should people best behave? Give up and accept exile from their former selves and lives? Or carry on as nearly "usual" as is possible for as long as is possible – perhaps benefitting from an extra level of clarity and understanding from those around them? In retrospect, I should have shoved Mum into the back of that camper van and let her take her chances of a new adventure in the Welsh hills. Instead, I mugged up Aricept and talked to the GP and she stood out on the grass in the middle of the "charity" sheltered housing complex and howled. It wasn't very long before the warden was calling the police and beginning the procedures to move her out.

The GP was more helpful. He'd already advised Mum that walking every day was the best thing to do and when I grizzled to him about how awful she was at the end of any special occasion: "Like a toddler after a party," I said, "throwing a tantrum in the evening when everyone has been doing their best for them all day long," he answered, "Yes – but you wouldn't not give your toddler a party, would you?" Six years on, now that she is more physically as well as mentally frail, I realise our approach needs to be a little more nuanced but at the time I felt that he was speaking in a language I could understand. He also said that the best that I could hope for was an "event" that would carry Mum off swiftly and painlessly. I don't think that's going to happen. I think we're in for the long haul – the full, unexpurgated Alzheimer's experience.

Margery experimented with several alternative titles and subtitles for *The Relay. Beloved Old Age – and How to Cope With It* was one of them. Another was *The Importance of the Family in the Practical Care and Protection of the Old in the New Society*. Her book is intended as a practical guide for families, though it extends the concept well beyond its usual limits. Margery's grasp of the interrelationship of body and mind ("the effects of physical trouble on the mental and emotional constitution") is sure. Others of us who are novices in the care of the old have had to learn rather sharply about the fragile balance of the elderly constitution and the ease with which it can be upset. We have to remember not to interpret personally things which are in fact medical. "Before deciding that an old person is 'impossible' it is as well to give one's mind to every aspect of his physical condition."

I used to think that old people's sensations were somehow

dulled, probably because many of them don't hear or see or smell so well. I've had to recognise that Mum's nonagenarian sense of touch is super-sensitive, as is her response to pain. I've only to spot a blister on her little toe and I'm racing for the First Aid cupboard to avert emotional upset. "You want me to sit on *this*?" she asks incredulously, indicating the cold, hard, toilet seat. I've found myself reflecting back to the combination of skin sensitivity and howling distress of a new baby and I wish I'd taken more trouble over those small, cossetting, nappy-warming details then.

One of the reasons that many medical professionals are glad to work with families is simple practicality. Someone with dementia (or any frail older person) may find it difficult to analyse their physical discomfort or communicate it other than through their behaviour. My friend Jo, a dementia nurse, shared an anecdote of a patient who suddenly began shouting at her daughter in Arabic. The daughter assured Jo that this was completely out of character: her mother was normally affectionate towards her and their usual language was English. Jo (a dementia daughter herself) diagnosed pain and sure enough, when analgesics were administered, loving family relationships were immediately re-established and speech returned to English. The involvement of that daughter had been the litmus which had made comprehension and then treatment possible.

In the spring of 1960, when Grace Russell came to share the bungalow with her cousin Maud, her dementia was already well advanced.[16] Margery's diary is generally uninformative about this period but the few comments in the weeks immediately after Grace's arrival record that Grace and

16 Grace Russell (née Allingham) 1871-1961.

Maud were "quarrelling" and "playing the goat", that Joyce was "having a time with them" and was "exhausted". Margery mentions a "hell of a set-out" at the Forge and the departure of the first live-in carer. A new carer arrived (described elsewhere as a psychiatric nurse) and "seems to think that we don't know what we've got hold of in Grace."

Cousin Grace, eccentric, generous and always previously ready to open her own home to other family members in need, was a former chorus girl. "At 89, Aunt Grace (a descendent of Princess Pocohontas on her mother's side, or so it is believed) just won't have it that anyone has died and we are constantly being instructed to prepare for visits from either of her husbands (both deceased), Papa (Granny's older brother) or the whole cast of *Floradora* with whom she appeared nightly in 1889."[17] Once installed in the Forge cottage, Grace could look out of her window at the pub across the square, convinced it was a theatre running regular evening performances, and no-one would contradict her. Unfortunately, she was also ready to shin out of that window and beg a lift to get herself back to London to make her own appearances. Grace, said Margery, kept them "from being ever exactly placid." Joyce remembered a surprising gaiety and humour as an intrinsic part of this period but also the worry, responsibility and tiredness. She supported the live-in carer and Margery supported her.

Well-planned care of one's "own old people" is more than a humanitarian response to a shipwreck; it is a complex and mutually beneficial process of handover and inheritance. Or so says *The Relay* and I am exploring its truth. It can cement family relationships or it can blow them apart. Margery and Joyce appear to have coped with Grace's dementia with the

17 MA to Isabelle Taylor (letter 29.8.1960).

same matter-of fact acceptance they extended towards Maud's depression and their mother's mischief-making tongue. This was a time, wrote Margery (after it was over) in which they received as much as they gave. The experience had enhanced her understanding of herself, her own identity, place in the world and possible future. Professionally she believed that "all sincere authors should be psychoanalysing themselves all the time" and was adept at transforming the experiences of her life into material for her art.[18] Despite its apparently limited scope, *The Importance of the Family in the Practical Care and Protection of the Old in the New Society* develops inevitably towards a meaning-of-life book.

Dementia is an illness that would be fascinating if it wasn't so upsetting. No two cases are the same as no two minds are the same. My mother's struggling brain blurs boundaries between perceptions. It experiences delusion, overturns chronology, confabulates. The process of listening and responding, reassuring, disentangling – following the ingenious meanders of a mind that has gone off-piste – can be rich in unexpected insights and connections. It can also be distressing and frustrating. The logic is emotional: events and observations morph into one another in dreamlike sequences (when they are not nightmares). Margery had always been interested in the paranormal potential of the mind: I wonder what she made of Cousin Grace's condition.

After Grace died, the last of the three relatives, Margery finally completed her long-drawn-out and overdue novel *The China Governess* and then wrote *The Mind Readers* in a creative burst. And, as she completed its final chapters, she

18 During the period that the old ladies were living in the Forge Margery was writing *The China Governess*, a novel particularly interested in inherited family characteristics.

wrote *The Relay* too.[19] *The Mind Readers* is probably the oddest of all her detective novels. In a genre that had historically prided itself on its appeal to ratiocination, it is defiantly more interested in "feels" than in thoughts. Apart from a passing reference to the use of a therapeutic activity (in this case button-sorting) to help recovery from delirium, there is nothing specifically to connect the book with observation of dementia. All one can say is that Margery is brimming with creative excitement and her subject is the emotional workings of the brain. *The Mind Readers* divides her admirers. Many (including Pip, her husband) dislike it intensely but Margery herself saw it as a new beginning and was excited by it. "One takes a great risk by being intelligible I always feel."[20]

No-one is going to take on the care of a person with dementia – or anyone else in the last phase of their life – for the sake of artistic self-development. Yet I begin to accept that my own mind has to become more flexible as I struggle to follow the sequence of my mother's thoughts. It's more than the misplacing of language; listening to Mum makes me conscious, somehow, of the different areas of the brain (the more and less damaged, currently) and how little I understand about its functioning. I find myself fascinated by theories of neuro-plasticity and brain regeneration as I observe how her ability to speak grammatically returns as we sit quietly on her sofa talking. Too often, when I arrive, she is monosyllabic, unable to use conjunctions, referring to herself as "me" not "I" – talking like a baby, in fact. But the habit of conversation is deeply ingrained in her and imperceptibly as we sit there,

19 *The Mind Readers* was with Graham Watson MA's British agent in October 1964: *The Relay* followed in November.

20 Letter to Paul Reynolds, MA's American agent, 16.6.1965.

holding hands, sipping water and looking towards that essential window, the patterns of language reassert themselves – and with them the ability to think more clearly. Or so it seems to me, in my mother's case.

Dementia is "more than just memory loss"[21], as all of us discover when we experience this illness – and, conversely, we also discover how much memory means, how fundamentally it underpins what we experience as person-hood. The extra effort I must make, now, to remember on my mother's behalf what she was like and the things she has experienced and could do, is transferring scraps of her identity across to me while she is still here. "I'd often heard that the personality crystallises after death," says one of Margery's characters in *The Mind Readers*, "but it had never registered on me before". Dementia is a dying of the mind: this process of crystallisation may perhaps start early, as we notice the abilities that have gone missing. The experience of dementia is different for us all however. I am speaking only for myself when I say that the patchiness with which Mum is losing mental functions sharpens my awareness of them. I sometimes feel that I must catch what I can before it's gone.

One of Mum's great qualities, I now realise, has been her ability to absorb herself in a project. I remember the relief I felt as a child when she began learning music as a way out of post-natal depression. It was her lifeline for years – and therefore ours too. She practised so intelligently and assiduously and achieved a great deal: gained a diploma, became a teacher, performed in concerts. But it was the learning, not the achieving, that mattered. Later she learned languages,

21 *Dementia: More Than Just Memory Loss*, published March 2016 by the Older People's Commissioner for Wales.

immersed herself in understanding the capabilities of her dog, bought herself a pony for her seventieth birthday then became fascinated by equine psychology as well as basic pony-care. This is all forgotten now and it is heartbreaking that even the smallest independent scheme is now completely out of reach. She therefore longs to do things "together". (That word itself has become a prop.) We spent a particularly happy afternoon before Christmas with me sitting on the floor writing cards and her folding a letter to go inside them. With intense concentration she could manage a single fold: two was beyond her. She wasn't exactly planting the roundel or playing the air but it was a very successful day.

One of the additional cruelties of dementia is forgetting how much has already been forgotten. Mum is currently entranced by the colours of the flowers on her window ledge and in the little strip of border we have commandeered outside. I left her, a few weeks ago, stubbornly determined to write a list of all the flower names and the names of the family members who had given them to her. She insisted that I provide her with pen and paper and words that she could copy. Probably I shouldn't have complied. She had, of course, forgotten that she can no longer read or write. But she was so happy sitting there assuring me that she "wasn't going to start the project yet" but would "just be busy making plans" as to how she was going to do it.

Saying goodbye is often hard. I feel the emptiness flood back into her room. We try to leave her holding something – a hot water bottle, her teddy, a bowl of custard – and we promise her that the next person (with a name) will be here soon. We point at the large clear clock, willing her to understand – or at least to trust us. If our reassurance doesn't work she will be out in the corridor searching, frantically wondering where she is and why she has been abandoned "in this great empty place". I have to go. I have other things that I need to do. I too have projects tugging at my mind. I recall Margery's advice not to "hold up my own sprint".

Mum knows this too and worries that I am spending too much time with her. She worries for Francis too and for our relationship and for my work. But I have become essential and she says so again and again. When the evenings are bad she hates me for leaving and is jealous that I have another home. She can play on my emotions, push me away whilst longing for me to remain. In her former life she was often glad to say goodbye: she regularly insisted that she didn't want people with her all the time; that she needed solitude for her own projects. I realise, now, how alike we are.

The day I left Mum projecting her list of flower names and donors was a good departure. She was not afraid to be alone, she waved me away, eager to get on with her plan. We have learned, during this winter, that we must not leave her by herself for more than an hour during the day – and that is frequently too long. By the time our friend Claudia Myatt arrived, Mum was in despair. She had realised, once again, that she has forgotten how to write. I wondered for how much of that intervening time she had remained confident and happy in the anticipation of her project before she discovered what I already knew, that a list, names, were of all things the most completely out of her reach. I should have managed it differently but I'm not sure how.

Claudia salvaged what she could. She picked up the pen and helped Mum practise writing her name. She reassured her that this was something that she could learn and we would all help. It could be a project in itself. But the tragic fact remains that it is learning, which was the joy of my mother's life and her particular skill, that is now completely beyond her. It sometimes seems that the more one repeats and "practises", the less she is able to do. Her mind tires. However valiantly she tries – and I applaud her brave spirit – dementia is an unlearning. The tide of her life has turned and this is the inexorable ebb. Swim against it, or row, as hard as ever we can, finally she will be swept out to sea. I will try to take comfort from the truth of Margery's perception that as Mum loses the knowledge of herself, it can be handed across to me and to the others, like Claudia, who are responding to her inexpressible Mayday.

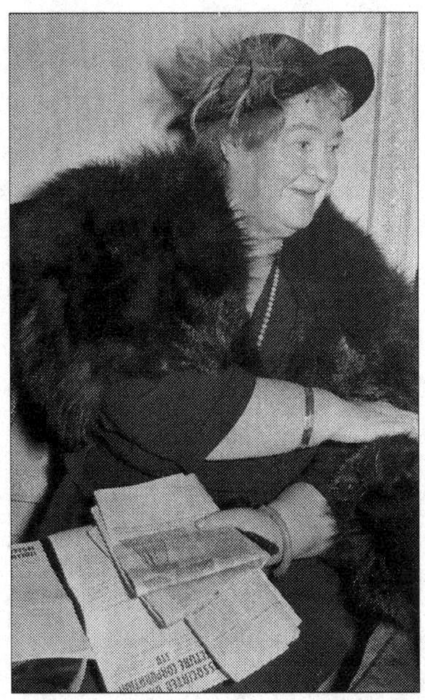

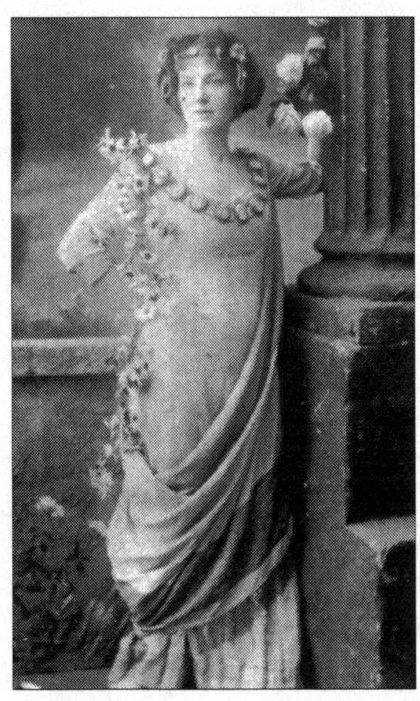

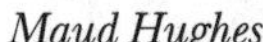

Maud Hughes

Grace Russell

Nowhere as bad as it looks
Margery Allingham

Probably the very first thing to be said about age is that it is nowhere as bad as it looks. So many modern commentators appear to take one scarified glance at a group of old people, superimpose in their mind's eye their own idealised elderly countenance and then break into wails of angry pity.

It is significant that to children and other old people the appearance of old age is reassuring rather than ugly. It is only to the middle years that its mere look is so particularly distressing. There is today a fashion for lightweight satire on the thoughts of old people. In fact, the thoughts of the old are remarkably like their own thoughts at any other age and if there were no looking-glasses a great many people would never dream that they were old. They might think they felt somewhat tired, or somewhat bored and inadequate, but no more so than they might well remember feeling at any other time, especially in puberty. Once seen, however, the cat is out of the bag. A portrait of any tired woman in her eighties, taken in an off moment when seated before an empty grate, can bring tears of dismay to most middle-aged eyes.

There is a popular fallacy about the old being fond of children; many of the old believe it themselves. "Now I am old I must be fond of children. How odd that I dread them so!" The theory is a sentimentalised, pre-digested, cheap version of the Relay take-over itself. The fact is that people who like children in youth and middle-age will like them still, even when they are old. But they are often wearied by them for physical reasons. The child drinks in life and the old person has little to give. Sometimes a friendship grows up between two people who are at the toddler stage – one old and one young. It can be a very strong bond, charming to watch. It is based on an absolute understanding of mutual disabilities; but at almost no other stage do the two meet as a matter of course.

Then there is the question of loneliness. The old look lonely. As they sit on the public seat, or by the window staring blankly at the street, or in bed gazing up at the ceiling, the spectacle which they present is of tragic solitude. But so, to an uninhibited seventeen-year-old, do all the people who sit in first-class railway carriages. The old certainly glance up eagerly when one addresses them and they like to talk until they get tired, but they are not a strange breed of lonely animals. They are preoccupied, ordinary people who are going somewhere, and they are on the emotional look-out for certain younger people, some of them strangers, to whom they are instinctively anxious to impart some small particular thing. Of course they tell the same things to everybody but do you plant one lettuce seed?

Loneliness in old age is no more than loneliness at any other time. Nor does living a long while turn the person who has eaten, slept and worked virtually alone for years into a gregarious old jolly-bird anxious to chirp his last in concert. I am not advocating solitary confinement, but no one is lonelier than a forsaken lover in a football crowd and if one has lived as one of a couple one will be lonely living alone.

Loneliness is not the thing that worries the old most, even if it is what the young find so guilt-provoking about their appearance. The thing that upsets the old most is being interrupted in their curious, secret and instinctive preparations during which they need care and protection and, from time to time, certain visitors, sometimes many. From the point of view of the heirs it is the break in the family continuity which must be avoided.

The habit of combining a reluctance to grow old oneself (a very healthy instinct) with ignorance of the facts of the subject may account for much of the quite unnatural terror connected with it. A great many otherwise normal people do refuse to face the fact of oncoming age either in themselves or in their nearest elders. They keep the possibility lying in the back of their minds like a time-bomb where it becomes more and more of a menace as its tick becomes louder. Yet these same people prepare for winter with the busy contentment of squirrels. Men and women seated on a warm bench in July can permit their thoughts to wander luxuriously to central heating, Christmas pudding and fur coats and can even contemplate biting winds and chapped hands without dread. Yet at the first whisper of the word age their minds tend to panic and their thoughts to crystallise into a single series of paralysed queries: "What shall I do when Dad…? When Mother…? When Auntie…? When Bill's mother…? When, oh God, when he…? When I…!"

We live in an age which has been brought up to believe that what is unpleasant is more likely to be true than what is not. In practice this generalisation is pure nonsense and it does not take much living before one comes to recognise it as one of those specious pieces of rhetoric like Mark Antony's "The evil that men do lives after them; the good is oft interred with their bones" which nobody, least of all the speaker, was ever expected to believe, but which sounds witty and provocative. The false prophets who preached cynicism to my father's generation had

their tongues in their cheeks. After a period when it was the fashion to pretend that everything was for the best in the best of all possible worlds it was a refreshing change, they found, to present the converse – if only because it was so shocking to a generation grown stupid with success.

Nowadays the false premise has presumably been rejected, since the young people who are buying their entire civilisation on mortgage, and gaily tying themselves down to repay at high rates of interest for the next thirty years, cannot be contemplating an endless line of broken marriages, ungrateful and delinquent children, disease, recession and the end of love, whatever they like to see in their theatres. In this modern world, which has decided not to go to blazes after all and is entirely new in that we have at last discovered that it is possible for everybody to be well off at the same time, it is still madness to be too casual to collect one's inheritance. It is not only the money, which anyone can afford to throw away – though even that is capital and should belong to the future. All the rest – the skills, the information about oneself and particularly the thing which the ancients so loosely called "the Blessing" (which is the unseen yet very definite thing which Jacob pushed in front of Esau to collect from his father) – those are vital and belong not only to oneself but to one's heirs.

The Blessing is the Field Marshal's baton among the rest, each person's own version of command. Thus, each old person only gives it to one young person. This, it would seem, is not necessarily the one he loves the best but the one most like himself who is there to receive it. It is as if he appears to say: "You are me as well as yourself. Certain of my emotional responsibilities have become yours. My half-finished business is yours and my rewards – anything to come – will be yours and

your heir's." As with every other legacy this is never pure jam in practice. Sometimes it proves bitter. Having inherited, one finds that one is fulfilling an ambition not one's own, righting a wrong one did not do, caring for something one would never have thought to care for before and which appears to be pure trouble until one discovers the life in it.

I am well aware that this is one of those statements which are like those about the existence of God or the shape of the Earth. It either strikes one as utterly and absurdly extraordinary or so obvious and well known that it hardly bears making. I put it here as a track-mark only. The people who know it do not need to be told again and the people who do know it will not learn it by reading.

How conscious is all this bequeathing and inheriting? It depends. Growing old is a part of life just as childhood was; how conscious were you of taking things in when you were a child? The chances are you are just about as conscious of giving them out again, amended, when you are old. Sooner or later the biologists and the psychologists will get together and make the process clearer and more dull. They still have a long way to go. However, it does matter. That is the one thing that the principal heir must steel himself to remember now, as far as we have got in this curious prefabricated civilisation.

Although only a few of the bequests seem to be material, and however negligible or unfair they may appear at the time, making sure that the right person receives the right thing, be it a ring or a recipe, a block of shares or a sense of debt to some family of whom one has never heard, it really is important because that is what the utterly fascinating performance is all about. Fozzle it, or consider it a duty when it is a privilege and so degrade it, and one does oneself and one's heirs a great disservice.

I had not intended to mention the unfairness but of course it always appears to be there because of the size of the operation. This is one of those things one needs a lifetime to express, but I can best indicate what I mean by saying that sometimes at an auction sale we think that our bid has covered a table-load of loot whereas, when it comes to it, we find that our purchase was the bird-cage and banjo only, and the elephant tusks had gone to the startled man standing beside us. It is not a mistake or a swindle; "his name was on them" as the soldiers say.

What appears to be required of the heir is for him to arrange the absorption of the old person back into the family where all that is going to remain of him here must be preserved. However it is managed, whatever it involves, however tedious the details, that is the necessity. The part of his personality or his programme which belongs to this world and is going to remain on it must be absorbed, and in nine cases out of ten that proves to be the thing the old person is really worrying about however clumsily he puts it. He wishes to impress himself upon certain people and to make certain of his heir. This ruined word "heir" is the true one and must be used here for clarity, even if it is lightened with that touch of self-derision which this era uses as a breastplate.

I mention this because so often the sacrifice which the younger person makes, and the personal inconvenience which he suffers, is all devoted to providing the things which seem least appreciated by the older person. It is when this is realised that the damaging things are said and done and the process of take-over is held up.

Probably the most individual item in each handover is the correct moment for it to begin. In nearly every case this is the unknown quantity. When the old person wants to move is the right time. As a rule this is usually decided by a crisis. A lease falls in, a landlady rebels, a *pension* "regrets", a fall occurs, an illness makes it necessary or an old companion is no longer there. At any rate, whatever it may be, it is an enormous asset to the younger people if they have made at least some rough mental provision for the emergency. One is seldom on one's toes waiting when the letter arrives, or more often, the phone rings. I suppose this is flashpoint; this is the moment when the balloon can go up in the most level-headed of households, and no emergency is made any more bearable by a thundering emotional upheaval at the outset, And yet "too soon" is, I sincerely believe, worse than "too late".

It is at one of these points, the penultimate moment before the "let-go", that one younger person realises that this is his cue and the take-over begins its run. It is seldom as easy as it sounds. Modern life is remarkably full. We have to plan for Christmas when returning from holiday at midsummer, and for next year's trip abroad as we take down the holly. It is because of this that the important developments in life are sometimes in danger of passing us by altogether. There are always situations in which one feels one's hands are tied, however this is one of the few occasions when a fight for one's personal right seems inevitable. Obedient dependence on the convenience of one's contemporaries is all very well but one must not forget to survive. This is personal and private and exactly as important in one's own story as one's marriage or the birth of one's child.

For the old person, if he moves house or merely takes a new boss into his own home, it must be a moment of "let-go". He may still have complete control of all his affairs and they may be still a deadly secret but he has had to make a change. Age has forced him to make an adjustment and even among people who are almost still at their best it is a difficult manoeuvre. Concessions on both sides, which neither had intended to make, are needed. These produce, conversely, little unexpected patches of mutual agreement and flashes of relief. To get off on the right foot it must also be a moment of truth.

Lest I make too much of this, perhaps I should mention that in my grandmother's case, when she was already nearly ninety and had given up her independence long before, she was evacuated one summer's day under the threat of Hitler's invasion and arrived in the house when I was alone and rather frightened. She was used to living in other people's homes and had no worries and no possessions. She looked with delight at the bed prepared for her and said: "Well, here we are! Now is there anything I mustn't do?" And I said, knowing all about her from childhood: "Well, darling, you know how you like to send people bits of news in your letters? Please never, never pick up a letter to me which you may find lying about and copy it out and send it to anybody at all, not even to the cousins in Canada, nor to Mama, nor Maud, nor anybody at all."[22] And she said, "All right, dear, if you say so, but we always used to do it long ago and people do like to hear about one. But if you say so, I won't." And I said, "All right, darling, God bless. See you in the morning." She kept her word and never did; not even the interesting ones from the bank manager beginning "Unless".

The moment, therefore, has to be taken when it comes; the whole thing is natural and therefore erratic. Like birth it can be induced but is better not.

22 Emily Jane Hughes's only son, Walter, had been killed at Ypres in 1915. He had previously emigrated to Canada, married and started a family.

"It can be induced but is better not"?
Julia Jones

Margery had spent the previous twenty-two years avoiding giving a home to her mother.[23] The days after Herbert Allingham's death in 1936 had been traumatic. Margery had found herself promising her father, whom she loved, that she would look after her mother, whom she had rarely liked. Em had already moved into Margery's house at Tolleshunt D'Arcy to be near the Colchester hospital for visiting. There were rows and dramatic scenes. Margery's husband, Pip Youngman Carter, decamped to London and Margery's grief for her father was horribly intensified by her mother's behaviour. After the funeral Cousin Grace at Pope's Hall stepped in and invited Em to stay with her – as long as there was a little money available to pay for her keep.

In 1936 Em Allingham was not old. She was in her later fifties, a strong and resourceful personality. After her time at Pope's Hall she found herself a job on Foulness Island as a housekeeper to a vicar whose wife was in an asylum. This developed into a relationship which lasted several years. When it ended Em moved about, sometimes staying with relatives, often living in lodgings or small hotels. Her pension was discreetly supplemented by Margery who used a lawyer to manage this. Em's own mother, Emily Jane, who had been living with Margery died in 1952 and in 1951 D'Arcy House had become fully Margery's property, *not* her

23 Emily Allingham (née Hughes) 1879-1960.

husband's. It was a big house with plenty of room for guests.

By the early 1950s Em Allingham was in her seventies but there were new reasons why her emotionally disruptive presence at D'Arcy House would have been just as intolerable as it had proved in 1936. Margery's marriage was in trouble, her mental and physical health was precarious and she was digging deep into herself to produce not only major novels but additional novellas and short stories in an attempt to keep ahead of an increasingly desperate financial situation. Both she and Pip had a relatively high public profile (he was deputy editor of the *Tatler*) and Margery was determined that there should be no hint of hidden difficulties. Successful authoress, beautiful house, happy marriage – these were more than props to her self-esteem, she believed they were essential business assets. Her mother would have had no hesitation in announcing the flaws. Margery's friend Mary Orr, recipient of much kindness, remembers being taken aside by Em and told, "Margery doesn't do it because she likes you, you know. She just likes to see herself being generous."[24]

Everyone has their reasons for not doing what they don't want to do. One of *The Relay* messages to which I cling is: "Old people can take lives without meaning to. It is up to everyone to protect his own". When my mother, in her eighties, became increasingly unhappy and unsettled in her pretty cottage near my brother and sister-in-law, I wondered desperately whether I should reorganise my home to take her in. Caring is a relationship-based activity and our relationship had hit an all-time low. Being with her then (before dementia was diagnosed) was like living on a bubbling volcano. Francis had been shouted at, the children harangued and as a consequence

24 Quoted in *The Adventures of Margery Allingham*, Julia Jones (Golden Duck 2009).

she and I had had the most damaging arguments of our lives.

I found other reasons for my reluctance. Our house is even more isolated than the cottage she was leaving. There is no public transport and she was no longer able to drive. Joining us at that point would have entailed the complete loss of her independence – and ours. Wherever she had wanted to go, we would have to take her. If we were away, she would be grounded. I could not quite see how any of us would survive the experience. I was profoundly relieved when she said she would like to move back to the small town near the River Deben where she had lived in the first years of marriage and where we had all been born. She could walk everywhere, catch trains, meet other people and continue to manage her own life. It was not yet the Mayday. Or so I hoped.

By 1958 when Margery finally accepted that her mother was desperate – Em was suffering falls, her bones had become brittle – her domestic situation had altered once again. Pip was living at home more often than in London, they had reorganised their financial affairs and were beginning to work together again. Margery was reassured and encouraged by this refreshment of their relationship. But Pip disliked Em. He disliked old age, ill-health, any form of vulnerability. Margery could so reasonably have decided not to jeopardise their rediscovered harmony by including her mother.

Instead she acted with assertiveness: "There are always situations in which one feels one's hands are tied, however this is one of the few occasions when a fight for one's personal right seems inevitable. Obedient dependence on the convenience of one's contemporaries is all very well but one must not forget to survive. This is personal and private and exactly as important in one's own story as one's marriage or the birth of one's child."

I had to read this statement more than once before I realised that the question of survival has been flipped. This paragraph does not, as I used casually to assume, refer to the everyday survival of the caring family member exhausted by the demands of the dependent oldie. The survival which is at stake here is the survival of the younger person's integrity. Margery is insisting that the right to care for one's elders is a personal right in itself, "exactly as important in one's own story as one's marriage or the birth of one's child." A successful hand-over from one generation to another is a defiance of mortality. It is put at risk by one's natural tendency to prioritise the expectations of one's own generation, partners, friends, employers.

Half a century earlier Margery had allowed herself to sacrifice her potential for motherhood "to the convenience of her contemporaries". "Kid v car really" she had commented then. In the 1930s when she was at the biological age and the stage of life when it would have been natural to start a family, she was establishing her career. As her sense of power and dedication as a writer grew, so she became more certain that her Campion novels needed to be given "everything that I have". She had felt neglected as a child: she did not wish to be a neglectful mother. In material terms, also, her responsibility was to earn. She needed all her productive capacity to support not only Pip and their over-large house but the friends who came to live with them, the staff they employed, the guests who partied there.

It is difficult, still, to achieve the right balance between being an available, nurturing parent and an earner. It is no easier when choices have to be made between being an available nurturing carer and an earner. The word "carer" hadn't even entered the language in 1958. It's possible that Margery and Joyce accepted responsibility for Em and Maud and, later,

Grace, purely out of duty but the explanation in *The Relay* is far more proactive. Families should care for their older members at the end of their lives for their own sakes, not as a duty or even out of altruism. They should do it because they will gain from the reabsorption of those older people's experience and qualities back into the family pattern. This is their inheritance.

Margery's difficulties with language – specifically the words "inheritance" and "heir" – offer us thought-provoking challenge. Traditionally there has been little problem accepting that people will care for and attend on older relatives if they expect to gain money or property. For some there is also the motive of reward in heaven. What Margery is saying is different: people should assert their right to care for their elders – however inconvenient this may be to those closest to them – because of the definite personal benefits they can expect in their understanding of existence.

This may be an idea that is easier to endorse after the process is over. I have heard other ex-carers say that they do not regret the careers and the activities that they gave up for the sake of the person who needed them. They feel enriched in knowledge both about the person they looked after and about themselves. About life too? Many say they feel empowered.

For myself, I am sitting here feeling as disempowered as ever I did in early motherhood when I had work that I wanted (or needed) to do and my childcare arrangements collapsed. Mum has reached the stage of dementia where she cannot be left alone for long. Margery's concept of an old person being intent on their "curious secret journey" depends, I think, on the mind and body remaining in step with each other. This is not our situation now. Mum has lost her way. She is lonely and frightened. Each day is therefore divided into three shifts.

On Tuesdays, Fridays, Sundays I willingly do all three, with additional "drop-ins" on the other days to ensure she sees me regularly. "Just passing, Mum, thought I'd drop in and say hello". It's an attempt to make her "extra care" flat feel like any ordinary home in the community where family and friends come in and out – but with an underlying pattern of routine that is intended to help her feel safe and well-orientated. That's the theory, anyway. When Mum isn't in a good frame of mind her flat is a "dump", a "prison". "You mean I have to stay here till I die?" "Run away, run away!"

There are usually two days in the week when I don't do any caring at all. I stay at home and work or I accept invitations to meetings, conferences – pleasure even. I could go sailing on those days. Visit the children or grandchildren. Loll around with Francis. Check whether I still have friends. Write a story! But, as every parent knows (and most rota managers too), when everyone else on the team is ill, on holiday or facing their own family crises, you are the person who will be filling in and whatever else you had planned will have to be postposed, abandoned or squashed into the dawn or midnight slot.

Take your toddler to work? I used to believe that I had my Mum-care days well sorted. She was so willing to enjoy whatever I was doing. I could organise my time round activities that I needed to do and which she could do with me. "Fitting-out", for example. That's the annual preparation of *Peter Duck* for the summer sailing season and usually takes place from the beginning of March. Ensconce mum on canvas chair with rug, thermos and plenty of biscuits. Add hot water bottle if necessary. Tell her regularly how well I'm getting on and how helpful it is to have her there and that's mutual happiness guaranteed.

Or so it used to be. Now that her mind is so clouded, so

exhausted by the daily struggle to survive, even fitting-out has lost most of its charm. She thinks she wants to do it but she is confused and fearful. If she sits too close she thinks the boat will fall on her: if she walks away she forgets where I am and feels lost. The noise in the yard frightens her: she is certain we are in the way of "the men". She gets tired and her bewilderment increases, painfully.

"You can't expect her to enter your reality any longer," the dementia nurse-consultant said firmly. "Even if it is something that she used to know and love. Now you must enter the world where she is. Anything else will disorientate her."

I have struggled to accept this concept. It sounds too much like the theory of "prescribed disengagement" when people diagnosed with dementia are routinely advised to (in effect) give up on their ordinary lives and wait to die.[25] Until very recently I've thought this was wrong in every way. I've felt certain that being busy, enjoying normal things together, hasn't just help me keep sane it has helped Mum too. Two years ago, aged eighty-nine she took up riding again, just gentle walks along a track with two cheerful girls and an understanding pony. That continued every Friday until this November, when somehow, for no very obvious reason, she didn't want to go anymore. Imperceptibly there has been a change: the cost of excitement has risen too high. I accept that I must be much more sensitive in adjusting my mind to hers – and moderating our activities as well. There are times when even listening to me read a poem or a *Swallows and Amazons* story is too much. We have passed some invisible tide gate.

Tomorrow is Saturday. The afternoon and evening care

25 The term was established by Australian writer and academic Kate Swaffer (www.kateswaffer.com).

shifts are already scheduled to be filled by me. I was happy enough – in the morning I was going get up early, sand the remainder of *Peter Duck's* hull below the waterline and, possibly, mend two dinghy fenders. Now Carol, the morning visitor, has called in sick. Carol is a professional. She's supremely reliable. I know she'd come if she could. That means the only person available to be there for Mum by 10.30am when the cheery "breakfast lassie" is gone, the morning phone-call time is over and she's sitting on her own in her flat, perhaps expectant, more likely depressed, is me.[26]

I don't WANT to spend the whole of Saturday in Mum's reality. Not when it's not one of the days that I've already mentally "given". It sounds like yet another stage on that damned journey that no-one ever asked me if I wanted to take. This does not feel equivalent to motherhood. I made a clear choice to have children – however naïve I was then about the effect they would have on my life. (I remember writing a detailed pre-birth timetable how I was going to manage my horses, my house and my first baby. No-one had warned me that he would demand a say in these arrangements. I howl with laughter now.) Tomorrow I need to do some fitting-out. I don't want to go to Deben View and sit on the sofa and modify our activities to suit wherever Mum is in her mind. Not all day.

But Mum is in a mental fog and drowning – or, as Claudia puts it "Her lines are loose and she's slipping away/ Drifting rudderless out of the bay".[27] I have to trust that *The Relay* is right. That all of this is a part of my life's experience; that it is comparable to parenthood and I will learn from it,

26 "Lassie" is Mum's word for all the carers who work at Deben View.

27 Song by Claudia Myatt written during the winter 2015-16. https://www.youtube.com/watch?v=ZqTe1ijzmF4&feature=youtu.be

as I did when my children were dependent on me and I will be glad of it, as I am of them. I must understand that this new unchosen form of caring is my inheritance and Mum's chance of immortality, through me.

I am clinging to this notion as if I am drowning too.

How can I survive tomorrow? *The Relay* is advising me not to "hold up my own sprint" and not to let Mum "take my life without knowing it" but dementia hasn't read the book. This evening Margery's messages feel about as dauntingly unrealistic as the 1970s theories of "superwoman" motherhood in which you ascend to the top of your profession whilst raising a brood of high-achieving, well-adjusted children, baking cookies, working out at the gym, looking effortlessly beautiful and being daringly imaginative in bed.

I have emailed out a family SOS but with little hope. This is Friday. It's late; people will have made other arrangements for their Saturday mornings – like caring for their children, for instance. Then my brother Nick rings. He has a committee meeting in the morning but could divert to Mum's on his way home. Could I do some of my fitting-out tomorrow afternoon? Could I!!

Margery and Joyce did manage to "solve the problem" of caring for their three old ladies without destroying Margery's marriage, finishing her writing career or missing out on this essential part of their human experience. Joyce continued to develop her considerable administrative skills and found time for personal pleasure through her two working collie dogs. She and Margery became closer and more mutually dependent. And the first thing they achieved was to tackle the housing question.

Where is the old person to live?
Margery Allingham

The next important thing is, where is the old person to live? Ideally the answer to that is "near the family's most authoritative member but not on top of him". Near so that he can receive protection from all the things from which hitherto he has protected himself. Near enough for the younger people to absorb his experience and all the other freight of his life which he is preparing to leave behind, yet not so near that he interferes with the younger lives which have problems and pleasures of their own. When the early blooms are fading it does not follow that the new buds should be shaded.

Very often an old person conceives a plan which includes moving his nearest and dearest into his own somewhat unwieldy dwelling. Once having got them there he keeps them more or less in bondage with a cross between bribery and blackmail, both extremely well meant. This can produce the most frightful repercussions without either side quite understanding what is happening. Now is the time for imaginative and constructive thinking on both sides. The following story is typical: A young acquaintance of mine had an aunt who promised to give him her house if he would do it up and come and live in it with his wife and look after her. It was a very awkward house, in shocking repair, but because the young man felt a duty towards the old lady who had always been kind to him, and because she was fond of the place, he agreed. The old lady continued to live in her house in her own way, which became naturally more and more slovenly the more helpless she became. The wife, who was house-proud, was overworked, unhappy and frightened. Meanwhile the initial repair bill became enormous and there was still more and more essential work to do. The old lady dared not assist with this because she felt she needed all her money, which was not very much, to live on in case the young man cleared out and left her. So he borrowed his wife's money and the work was finished and the house became worth much more than before.

At this point, the old lady read a story in a newspaper about an elderly person who had made a deed of gift to a relation on exactly the same terms as those she was proposing herself. As soon as the deed had been signed, the relative was killed in a motor smash, his wife inherited and became dominated by a second husband and the old lady was left homeless. This depressing story made such an impression upon my acquaintance's aunt that she retracted her promise and decided to leave the young man her house in her Will. So the young man found himself living in a house which he did not like and on which his wife had spent all her money, while the old lady required more and more careful nursing and the overworked young wife became utterly exhausted.

Soon the old lady had to receive professional care in a special place and when at last, after the unhappy couple had lived in the house for five years – being unable to sell or let it, of course – and had paid the heavy nursing home bills, which they felt were their responsibility since they could not look after the old lady as they had promised, she died and they inherited. The increased value of the house on which they had spent so much money sent up the size of the estate, which was now taxed at a very much higher rate than it would formerly have been. They had to sell. The wife scarcely got her money back, the young man did not, and in the back of his mind he always felt that the old lady thought he had betrayed her trust by not seeing that she was nursed to the end in her own home.

However, the man who is faced with the prospect of taking his mother into his bandbox of a house where she will destroy the health, temper and comfort of a wife he adores is in a dreadful predicament. So also is the woman who is torn between her filial affection and her husband who needs her for himself and their own children. She struggles with her conflicting feelings and her husband may easily be turned against her by the double dose of her family's flavour which he observes in their own home atmosphere. This concentration of family personality is most noticeable to in-laws at these times and causes most of the friction which can be so destructive. Too much Smith at one time can be suffocating to a young Mrs Smith née Jones.

Then again a young man living in his own home in which he has established two entirely separate ménages, one for his young and one for his old family, should not be misled by: "She says there is no need to put in the extra front door because it won't be needed as soon as..." This is a false line of thought and unimaginative. "She" is going to be busy altering more than a front door. There are a few old people like Granny who trot along beside the new sprinter handing out batons like Santa Claus but they are rare. More often the following kinds of natural situations must arise and any one of them can upset either applecart: "If Mama has that nice woman to look after her, surely they can babysit?" "Couldn't we borrow that big room just for the wedding?" "Mama is bribing the children/ hired help/you!"

On the other hand, there can be a chorus from the old who are roosting in the homes of the young: "Oh, I'm comfortable but I have to have the radio as loud as this to hear it." "I rang because if someone is going out in that car, could they take me to see Henry?" "Of course I've sacked the woman! She insulted me. Someone else must get me to bed." "I have written to the Welfare Officer/Chief Constable/Pope. I want him to see this wash basin I've been given." "When the doctor/parson/relative/ absolutely anybody comes to this house, he comes to see ME." "I'm determined to pull my weight but I've had a little accident with the kitchen stove, dear…" "But I don't feel it's my house…" "I won't have help. I won't unlock the door," and so on.[28]

In an attempt to do their best for their elders most people in these modern days work out a compromise. They afford the guest house and mortgage the future. Or they pull every string and get a place in a public institution, which is not easy. Out of this situation the phenomenon of the Hostel for Old People has arisen. These unwieldy country houses, open to those who do not require nursing, are often submerged in greenery at the end of long drives; lost oases of silence and well-kept gloom. All of them, however faithfully managed, have the same curious atmosphere, which at best is boarding school and at worst is the Dustbin play.[29] One sees room after room of swaddled men and

28 "The idea of an old relative sitting comfortably and tidily in a corner of a modern suburban house is obviously unreal. A seat by the hearth in a mediaeval castle or fully staffed farmhouse, where like some precious pet in his basket, the old eyes can watch the sparks fly upwards, with people coming and going is one thing. A wheelchair huddled close to the radiator in one contemporary room, deserted and alone from 8am to 6pm and manifestly in the way when everyone returns home from work is asking too much of any old person or family." (in alternative *Relay* version)

29 Probably a reference to Samuel Beckett's *Endgame* (premiered Royal Court Theatre 1957).

women presenting an unmistakable picture of a long wait for nothing at all. The visiting relatives, seated wretchedly on the edge of their chairs as the tedious minutes loiter by, seem to be wondering if it is their own consciences they have called to placate. They try to make it up to the older person by car rides, by presents, by constant nagging thought and worry.

Whatever the fees for this kind of place and whatever the standard of comfort, the effect upon nine-tenths of the company is astonishingly the same. Their faces present a blank, proud, helpless "I-am-travelling-in-a-first-class-compartment-to-somewhere-I-don't-care-if-I-arrive-at" expression which is unmistakable and more depressing than anything else in the world. It is so usual that one begins to believe that it is the natural face of old age. Yet, one has only to talk to one's own old relative in such a place to find that, behind it, he is still himself, if with some new and alarming symptoms. The most usual of these are helpless resentment, bitter contempt for a society which has condemned a human being to limbo, maudlin self-pity or, in more refreshing cases, straightforward abuse of everything and everybody including oneself.

To make matters worse, whoever is paying, the cost is fantastically high. Very often the conscience-stricken relative is spending quite recklessly on the grumbler's presumed comfort. Also, he is expending the capital which he knows will be needed for his own sojourn in Crematorium View, or whatever the place is called. The general artificial segregation of the old is as dangerously unnatural as general artificial insemination and, in a way, rather like it. Integral pieces of human experience are by-passed and lost by both.

Although it is obviously a beneficial thing for us to look after our own old people the question which remains is often the terrifying one: Whose life? Yours or ours? It is here that the importance to the members of the dominant generation of understanding the temperaments of the older members of the family is not, perhaps, as obvious to us today as once it was. Nothing quite so vital can be lost for long. Sooner or later people will cease to wonder so anxiously how to keep alive and will go back to wondering why they want to do so.

At the risk of trying to teach a grandchild how to suck an egg perhaps I might point out that few people have proved more practical in the long run than Moses. His pronouncement that men should honour their fathers and mothers (presumably by thinking about them intelligently) was for the good reason he gave; that they gained thereby the longest view. As he indicated, this is the only way of getting the widest overall picture of life so that the general pattern of one's family story and one's own contribution to it can be seen. This cannot be the whole story, of course, but it is one aspect of our lives in the land that was given us, and goes quite a way to explain what on Earth we are doing.

As I have said the legacies or batons which the old pass to the young are not often very apparent. My grandmother lived with me during the war and through the almost worse period just after it. If she had not been there I should have left my post, which would have been a bad thing for me and many other people. I do not intend to list the benefits she conferred upon me but none of them were what is usually called material. For instance, I never knew she had a purse until she died and when at last it was unearthed it was seen to contain three pence and a platform ticket to Southend railway station. All were mouldy. She was not clever and she was not amusing but she was the most remarkable source of human peace and security I have ever known. The things I inherited from her were many and have made me happy and comfortable although I was not her main heiress.

However, when my sister and I were faced with the care of her niece and two daughters, the question of "whose survival?" arose again. I remember thinking when I was little more than a girl that I would give my parents anything except my life. In the forty years since then I have altered many of my hard-and-fast convictions but not that one. Old people sometimes take lives without noticing it. It is up to everybody to protect his own. There is, however, a tremendous element of proper pride involved in the situation which those who try to settle the question in a public welfare fashion, sometimes misunderstand. My father's dignity is my dignity: the respect due to my mother is the respect due to me. This is basic and indestructible. Dignity and respect are not to be thrown out of the window because no one has yet invented a mechanical nurse.

Well then, what was the answer for us? What were we to do? Here we were halfway through a great physical and social change, with everything happening faster than it used to do except for the process of growing old which alone takes longer than ever. Our own old people were all very strong, powerful, self-opinionated, egotistical women who did not want any help from anybody. We loved, respected and were very grateful to them all and had seen a great deal of them throughout our lives. I do not intend to make this a book of personal reminiscence but I would mention this and one or two other minor items because it is the easiest way of giving an illustration.

The three presented different types of problem – all fairly usual. Aunt Grace was marvellously active and marvellously senile. Aunt Maud was a power and an authority who had learned how to be popular by using her head; she was used to making money and spending it and getting her own way. Her first stroke embittered her and destroyed her will to make herself charming in exactly the same way as it stopped her running her office and managing her staff. Her friends said it had altered her personality and changed her temperament. Actually it had done no such thing but it had taken away her powers of using her skills to further her main desires, which had not altered. She wanted to go back to manage her office and her staff, and because she was no longer clever enough to do this, she sulked. A nursing home was out of the question for her for financial reasons.

Mama was supposed to be the most difficult of all. She was the person with whom everybody had, as they say now, a love-hate relationship. She was a charmer to strangers for the first few days and a terror to them ever after. She could be more entertaining than anyone I have ever met. An accomplished fairy-story-teller who, as she grew older, became less and less scrupulous about the trouble she caused by it. She was also one of those people who invariably cut off the bough on which they sit.

She had made up her mind that my husband's house, of which he was very fond and which he had purchased with his own patrimony, was morally hers because the man who had lived in it in her youth had promised to leave it to her.[30] For the last twenty years of her life her unswerving determination was to come and live in it as soon as her own mother died and made room for her. At which time she meant, as she was never tired of explaining, to take over the household and turn it into

30 When Dr Salter, the previous owner of D'Arcy House died and left the house to his business partner, Em Allingham's disappointment was such that it triggered a nervous breakdown. In 1935 a loan negotiated by Herbert Allingham, together with a gift in lieu of legacy from Pip's mother Lilian Carter, had enabled the young couple to buy the house together. After their marital crisis of 1951 the house had been made over entirely to her.

the Edwardian dream which she had conceived when she first saw the building. The practical aspect of anything she wanted to do had never bothered her and it was astonishing how much she achieved without considering it; but not, of course, how apprehensive this made everybody else.

I mention these three cases because together they embrace many of the most common types of modern "difficult" relatives. The fact that we could see them all converging on us together and had to give our minds to this in the way that people who have had a typhoon warning must, is the only unusual element. As a rule people muddle through somehow, but often somebody gets hurt and the experience is seldom pleasant or satisfactory. In our case the prospect seemed impossible if we aimed to survive.

On the death of my grandmother, the renewed interest of my mother in my husband's home was expressed in her restlessness as she moved from one *pension* to another, a heart-breaking and unhappy figure.[31] The habit formed by Aunt Maud of spending every other weekend with us, so that she could be "cleaned up" and "put straight" for the next fortnight's dedicated and influential but, by the new standards, not very well-paid work, brought the subject closer and closer. It was Aunt Maud's doctor's solemn warning, and his clinical description of life and its requirements after a major stroke, which made us broach the matter seriously, at least to each other. Aunt Maud was already old enough to be no longer very interested. She disbelieved the doctor and thought his prognosis worse than death and therefore merely unkind.

31 There is a thick file of letters from Em to Margery dating from this period. They are overtly affectionate but tell a tale of many little hurts and squabbles. "I've always found life difficult," she writes revealingly, "and I realise all you children have as well." (25.4.1954)

"Worse than death"?
Julia Jones

Was it the prospect of permanently impaired cognition that so appalled Maud Hughes? The damage done to the brain by a major stroke can be ruthless in its removal of intellectual as well physical functioning. Maud suffered a second stroke while she lived in the Forge Cottage but survived another eight months: "a long and miserable illness," commented Margery afterwards. The unpredictable series of blocks and bursts and mini-strokes that are labelled vascular dementia can take years to achieve their similarly destructive result. Vascular dementia is the second most common form of these degenerative brain diseases, the first being Alzheimer's, and there are many others. Today we are more frightened of dementia than we are of age.[32] It is progressive, terminal and currently incurable, the most common cause of death in women and second most common in men.

It is not only people without dementia who are afraid: people living with the illness are frequently terrified. Perhaps they are terrified all of the time, I don't know, I can only speak from my observation of and conversations with my mother. Before this period in our lives I might have assumed that people with impaired cognition were relatively unaware of their

32 In the 1960s life expectancy was 71 and rising and the population was 52 million. The fertility rate was 2.69 live births per woman and falling. In 2015 life expectancy was 81 and rising and the population 64.6 million. The fertility rate was 1.83 live births per woman and falling. There are 850,000 people living with dementia in the UK today, more than 47 million globally.

altered behaviour. I remember my grandmother asking the same questions, telling the same stories again again, She began to seem stupid, unresponsive, "gaga". [33] I have only a single bright and happy mental picture of her other than as a grim-faced old lady. I understand now that hers was the lion's face of Alzheimer's. At the time I thought it was because she was old. I soon began to treat her with politeness rather than love and I wish I could apologise. I don't think the adults around her understood her condition very well either. The places in which she lived her final years were terrible.

My godmother, married to my mother's oldest half-brother, fared better (I think). [34] Her illness was explicitly understood to be dementia and she spent about fourteen years in nursing homes before she died in 1990. My uncle, who had not been a perfect husband in other ways, visited her daily and devotedly and I am told that she never lost her charm and warmth of personality even in the final stages of non-recognition. Mum loved her and visited, though it was a long way away and things were not easy in her own life then. I use Aunt Ruth as an example to try to reassure Mum than she is not the only person who has this bewildering condition. Mum came home one day with an anecdote of her brother lifting a soup spoon to feed his wife and Ruth saying, "What*eve*r is that?" She was not frightened: simply amazed and curious. I can still make Mum laugh with that story even though I am using it to explain her own illness to her. "Is this the book then?" she asked a few days ago, lifting up the milk jug and waving it recklessly. The book, a particularly precious volume, loaned by a friend, was lying open and forgotten on her lap. When words go, things morph hopelessly together.

33 Edith Maud Jones (née Wilson) 1882-1971.

34 Ruth Scott (née Moorsom) c1904-1990.

Aunt Ruth is perhaps our equivalent to Margery's Granny, Emily Jane Hughes, loving and beloved and well adapted by her own qualities to meet almost any eventuality. Perhaps Nicci's father John Gerrard, who lived well for ten years after diagnosis of Alzheimer's, was also blessed by his own personality as well as the love and companionship of his wife and family. It's not that simple though. Nice people don't necessarily dement nicely. A friend was married to one of the gentlest and most sensitive people I have ever met. They were both musicians and theirs was a real love affair. He was a generation older than she was and when dementia overcame him he became dangerously violent and had to move into a secure facility. There he settled. My friend and their children visited regularly and the other three members of his string quartet came every month to make music for him.

Denis had been a Japanese prisoner of war and I'd always known he was one of the survivors of the building of the bridge over the River Kwai. I only thought, rather superficially, wow, and looked at him in awe. It wasn't until Mum and I went to his funeral and listened to the last of his former comrades speaking about their experience that I felt I had any understanding of the trauma they had suffered.[35] I also learned what the disabling of his hands through that period had meant for Denis as the pre-war possibilities of his career as a concert violinist ended. Too late I realised what fantastic inner bravery and self-control Denis had been exercising to achieve those decades of productive and happy life. Until dementia kicked away his coping skills.

My mother is a little younger than Denis and suffered

35 The speaker was Fergus Ankhorn. His (and Denis's) experience is recorded in *Captivity, Slavery and Survival as a Far East POW: the Conjuror on the River Kwai* Peter Fyans (Pen and Sword 2011).

differently as a result of the war. She too has lost the vital skills she has used all her life to keep the personal trauma at bay. There will be thousands of others, not necessarily of the wartime generation, who are left exposed by dementia to the terrible ghosts of their past.[36]

Maud Hughes had already been widowed more than ten years before her first stroke. When she lost her ability to work, she lost her identity. She had no children, she had very little money. Had it not been for Margery and Joyce (and, to some extent, their brother Phil) she might have ended her days in a Public Assistance Institution like my poor Granny. When Margery speaks of relatives "pulling every string (to) get a place in a public institution" I wonder whether that's what my father and uncle did. I can only assume that Granny's end was part of collateral damage in their own lives because – from my remembered perspective as an ignorant teenager – I think they should have been pulling every string to get her out.

My grandmother had been born in Whitby but her family's roots were further north towards the Scottish borders. She had been widowed early and had endured hard times in the 1930s agricultural depression. When her second son Jack was invalided out of the Navy in 1945 he bought a house on the River Deben and she lived there with him. I think they were good years. When my parents married they were just a few miles away and we were regularly in and out. I remember that Granny lived in a sunny ground floor room with French windows onto the garden. It was a big house: room for Uncle Jack's yacht design office as well as his expansive private life. When financial and other crises overwhelmed him in the later

36 *And Still the Music Plays: Stories of People with Dementia*, Graham Stokes (Hawker Publications 2010) mentions survivors of childhood abuse, for instance.

1960s he was forced to sell and he moved to a tiny, though exquisite, town house. Another triumph of the 1960s, the decriminalisation of homosexuality in 1967, meant that he could at last live openly with a partner.

There was, however no room for Granny. She went to a nursing home in Felixstowe and I remember her on the promenade tucked round with rugs, looking content and cared for. Presumably the money ran out there as well. Did my parents ever consider offering her a home with us? I suspect not. Probably Granny was too ill by then and there would have been other valid reasons. The places she was sent were called hospitals. The two I remember were both former workhouses, bleak, overcrowded and impersonal. When my mother moans about her spacious sheltered flat – "this dump" – where she is cared for by kind and thoughtful support workers and visited daily by family and friends, I sometimes picture my granny, in that long line of beds, never wearing her own nightie, bewildered and smelling of urine. Once or twice I've lost my temper and said so, but that's a waste of breath and quite unkind. Mum can't remember and there's nothing now that will change whatever went wrong then.

Our own choices have not been perfect. In my relief when Mum chose to move back to the town where we'd been born I minimised the question of distance – or rather I assumed it was a problem for us and our petrol bills but not for her. There was an initial bad choice of accommodation but after that I thought we had it right – as long as we remained determined to put in the miles. Mum's flat is "sheltered" and "extra care" – options that were not generally available in the mid-twentieth century. It has so much about it that is good but, despite all our efforts, she feels lonely and far away, even beside the river which she first discovered almost seventy years ago.

In the later stages of dementia, sheltered housing and extra care only works with assiduous input from family and friends. When I hear my mother's neighbour calling, "Help me, help me, help me," I wonder who can truly answer her. "Mum, Mum, Mum," she cries. I meet a brave old lady stomping the corridors. Her knees ache and she is blind. She is almost always lost and trying to find the way back to her flat. People walk with her willingly but she cannot settle there. She wants to go home. We sing "The Oak and the Ash and the Bonny Ivy Tree" as I help her up the stairs but there's no one left for her in the North Count*ree*. How has she washed up on this East Coast?

I notice Vickie, one of the carers, walking with her in the sunshine round the big garden. Vickie's mother also has dementia and lives miles away in Liverpool so Vickie has reorganised her working life to ensure she goes back to Liverpool regularly. So many professionals who work in health or social care are family carers themselves, out of hours. "I organised all the care for both my parents," says the housing association manager, "I made sure they lived and died in their own home – and they were in Pakistan. It was very tough but I am glad that I did it." One in three of us can expect to be carers in our lifetime.

People with dementia are much more likely than their contemporaries to be living in institutions yet, of all people, their need for individual understanding is greatest. Medicine can achieve so little: relationship is almost the only panacea. My mother goes out into that corridor and screams in her abandonment. She pleads to be taken "home". In fact, the best thing that has happened recently is that the housing association, together with a social worker and a dementia specialist nurse, have formally agreed with me that Mum is best staying where she is. She will not be pressurised to move out (as she was from the "charity" housing) and we will continue to look after her in partnership – to the end, I hope. But I don't yet know.

Yes, I wish that Deben View was physically closer to my house and, yes, I admire other people who have turned stables or cowsheds into delightful self-contained accommodation for their elderly relatives and, yes, perhaps we should have made a different decision earlier. But now, six years later, however bad these winter months have been, I am certain that any move elsewhere would bring calamity. Her disorientation when she is tired or upset can be extreme and terrifying. "I don't know where I am, Jul." "You're in your bed, Mum." Yet, most of the time, she recognises her sofa, a few pictures and the view from her window – even when she is trying to run away from them.

"You mean I have to stay here till I die?" she asks in horror. "Hope so," I answer bafflingly, knowing how few people die in their own beds and she still has hers. When Mum's GP told me that Deben View "let people die in there," I knew she was paying them a compliment. Too many doctors see frail and demented people in the last stages of their lives shipped out of their Homes to die in hospital. "Run away, run away," says Mum.

There is a radically abridged version of *The Relay* in Margery's archive written after she had spent a month in hospital during 1965: "No disgrace attaches to an old person dying at home under the care of the family doctor. Indeed it is better to die privately in one's home in familiar surroundings among people one knows than in hospital. The prayer of the aged is 'Lord now lettest thou thy servant depart in peace'. There is no professional merit in an old person dying with needle, transfusion set, catheters, defibrillator, heart lung machine and artificial kidney in place. Prolonged dying may ease a morbid conscience or feed a professional narcissism but to fill a patient's last hours in his world with pain and anguish is surely not good medical practice." Almost fifty years later the 2014 Reith lecturer, Atul Gawande, said very much the same.[37]

But once again I'm writing from my inexperience, guessing, but not knowing, how challenging those last, unimaginable stages may be. I make decisions but then I am uncertain. Is there any other way we can answer Mum's longing to come home other than doing all we can to bring home to her? And where is "home" anyway?

When I read Sally Magnusson's brilliant book *Where Memories Go* I felt despair.[38] Sally's mother Mamie Baird was living (and dying) with Alzheimer's. She was a widow but still in the house where she and her husband had been happy, still living with the twin sister who had made her home with them for many years. A full-time carer was employed and Mamie's three devoted daughters and her grandchildren set up a rota of family visits. Margery's ideal arrangements, as set out in *The Relay*, could not have been bettered. Yet still Mamie Baird pleaded to be allowed to go home.

Sometimes, when I listen to Mum it sounds as if home is in fact death or some pre-existing life. Home with God, perhaps? Many people assume it is the childhood home or place of birth. Home is "where the children are", says Margery. Sally Magnusson suggests home is the lost identity. If that is so, the case is hopeless.

It is hopeless, of course, yet perhaps there is something to be gained from *The Relay*'s idea of transference? Can identity can still be found through relationship when it has fled from

37 *Being Mortal: Medicine and What Matters in the End,* Atul Gawande (Metropolitan Books 2014).

38 *Where Memories Go: Why Dementia Changes Everything,* Sally Magnusson (Two Roads 2014)

any specific location? Margery writes: "What appears to be required of the heir is for him to arrange the absorption of the old person back into the family where all that is going to remain of him here must be preserved. However it is managed, whatever it involves, however tedious the details, that is the necessity." I think Magnusson and her family achieved this magnificently. Mamie Baird lives on in *Where Memories Go* and I'm going to hazard a guess that she lives on in their lives.[39] I hope to some point Mamie herself felt it as a comfort. Mum told me yesterday that she likes to feel "part of something." I believe that's the best we can do.

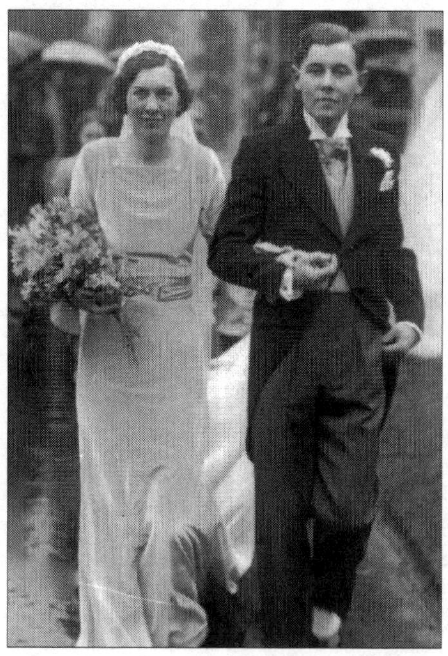

Ruth Moorsom and Anthony Scott on their wedding day at Harrow. They fell in love in the late 1920s when he was a schoolboy and she a housemaster's daughter. His devotion endured to the end of her life

39 Mamie Baird also lives through the music charity Playlist for Life.

The impossibility of my own and my sister's problem
Margery Allingham

The impossibility of my own and my sister's problem – with the latest news of Aunt Grace ominous – set us thinking very hard indeed. As one does if the position appears too much like disaster, we turned to speculating what would be the very best that could be done by us, for them and ourselves, if we could wave a magic wand and have every resource: a large room for two people with washroom, lavatory, kitchenette plus some other less elderly person's dwelling just off it, steady background heating which could be augmented in cold weather, and arrangements for airing the place without making it draughty. These were the essentials but we would like constant hot water, a washing machine, spin drier, a contrivance for privacy round the bed, storage space, venetian blinds, a view outside of something going on and not too much noise although not dead silence either, and the luxury of a glass porch or prefabricated sun room.

When I first considered this list it seemed a wild pipe-dream because I had no illusions about the second half of this "where to live" requirement. The second half is human. A self-contained flat or cottage is all very well but without human care it is little better than any other box.

To get the list of requirements perfectly clear in my mind I also made it in reverse. What were the items any old person did not want? To my astonishment the answer added up to almost everything else in the world except for a few strictly personal items. Once an old person has the essentials, his needs seem to be all negative and to become fewer as the process of age continues, as I had seen in slow-motion with grandmother. Peace, comfort, protection, accessibility to everybody wanted and none to those who are not. Care when needed and no restriction. That was almost everything. The really expensive things of life – change, fashion, travel, entertainment, kicks – were all of them in the out-tray, unneeded and unregretted.

The three human requirements were Protection, Companionship and Care. The last two can be synonymous but are much easier to arrange if they are kept quite separate.

Companionship is the thing the residential home or guest house attempts and does not manage to give. Two are company, but anything more is solitude again. An old husband and wife, two siblings, two friends, two contemporaries – or even two old enemies – are capable of living together in complete comfort if the room is large enough. They share the expenses, the gossip, the grumbles and, more often than one might expect, the hilarity. Two back each other up like contemporaries sharing a taxi. They may sometimes irritate each other but for those who are not deeply religious and whose last companions are not truly the angels, a second person is essential.

Obviously, this only applies to the old who are not sick. The great illnesses (and by these are not meant the normal healthy aftermath of strokes, broken bones, rheumatic and other chronic conditions) require the hospital beds with professional nursing and should have them. But the merely old simply want a quiet life at home where their younger people can keep them in the family picture as they jog along, only just out of the main stream. Another contemporary for companionship, then, and after that, service and care.

To get hold of human Care in this age of "everything-else-but" seems at first sight to be quite impossible. However, the question to ask oneself is, exactly what sort of "care" is needed for two old people, mobile or near mobile, living close to the authoritative protection of their nearest and dearest? The answer has two aspects: what they can be seen to need and what they say they need.

They can be seen to need interest in their welfare, considerate help with their goings to bed, gettings-up, washing and dressing. Their food prepared and served to them, their rooms kept clean, their laundry taken away dirty and brought back washed and aired. Their desires listened to and relayed, and the minor exasperations which are part of the story of becoming a little blind, a little absent-minded, tidied up without reproach. They also need someone within call almost all the time and this person must be able to defend herself lest she be turned into a recalcitrant slave. Besides this, at least twice a week, they need the services of a nurse for baths, nails, hair-dressing and that knowledgeable once-over which can tell at a glance whether it is a doctor or an aperient that is needed.

What they say they need are exactly the items listed above but concealed under almost every conceivable disguise: "a good north country landlady", "someone just like oneself (!)", "someone cheerful and not fussy", "someone who will bring the food and GO!", "a sensible person one would not mind asking to 'do things'", "a companion", "my daughter" – in fact, absolutely any woman of almost any age who will take the trouble to find out what is wanted and will make an honest effort to supply it. Arranging to get this sort of care can still be done if the approach is right.[40]

The requirements are simple but they are very strict and must be laid down beforehand and constantly adjusted and sympathetically observed, and this must be done not by the old person but by the young one. This last is a vital requirement and in nine cases out of ten will need help from the old person's intelligent solicitor to protect the young one should he be misunderstood. Providing care and its administration is one of the first responsibilities to be handed over in the Relay and nearly all the early failures are caused by one party funking it. A moment's thought will make it clear to the younger person why the appointment of the Care and her employment must be his own business.[41] The woman is not needed to represent him as son or head of the house but she is needed to do all those small services which members of the family would otherwise do themselves. The younger person alone must control this service and be responsible for it, for he alone can defend or control the old people if needs be.

The chief difficulty I anticipated at the time was the fact that the two relatives whom we foresaw living together had never liked each other very much. In practice that fact did not even emerge. The remark one so often hears and sometimes makes, "I would rather die alone than live with old so-and-so", belongs with the other common misstatements mentioned earlier. At forty, one never feels that one should be "put down"

40 The "head of the house" was always Margery but *The Relay* consistently attempts to persuade men that this is also their business. Margery once told her secretary Gloria Greci, "If you have to hold a man up, you may as well make sure you hold him up the right way."

41 The Care = the Help = the Chatelaine: Margery made different attempts to find the right word.

and when one is old one does not care who "old so-and-so" is as long as he is there, an ally in any common emergency which may arise to disturb one's changing existence and new task.

In practice, companions who are not related often disturb each other less then relatives do, because temperamental peculiarities are not then repeated and thus emphasised – or so it seems from the outside. At any rate, compatibility between the young people who are making the practical arrangements seem almost more important than between the older people involved.[42] Great social and educational differences themselves appear to matter little although, of course, the degree of sensitivity and civilised behaviour does, though less so than at any other time. This is no occasion for anybody to attempt to cure, say, snobbery in one person or to strive to instil a few social graces into another. The aim is not improvement but protection during a natural change of form, a process which must never be confused with any physical illness which may coincide with it.

The more thought given to these requirements before the moment arrives for some practical move to be made, the clearer the idea becomes. When it finally emerges and one sees it as a whole, it proves to be a familiar picture but translated into the modern idiom.

I hardly like to mention the term "dower house" because at first it sounds so wonderfully archaic and luxurious. Yet the name, like calling the family "the heir", is the correct one because it is the original answer to the original requirement. Our ancestors, who had a great deal of time for trial and error, conceived the idea of the dower house and it is well worth while examining its peculiarities. As one considers them, their

42 Forge Cottage was used for two other unrelated old people after Maud had died and Grace was there alone.

ingenuity emerges at once and one sees that dower houses were designed to fit the human heart and mind and that every natural need and weakness has been thought about earnestly. The aim has been to avoid just that kind of family trouble which one dreads, and which is likely to be most damaging in this period of renewal, when family solidarity is most needed.

For example, any dower house is smaller than the main house but it is of exactly the same tone and quality. It is readily accessible to the main house but it does not dominate it. It has its own front door, its own entity, and expects to entertain its own guests: any official has been invited to see Mother's own washbasin and not the one she has been given. Conversely, no one wants to borrow an old person's bedsitting room in someone else's house for any wedding. It does away at once with any resentable nonsense about "this attic", "outhouse" or "hen house down the garden".[43] It is smaller because it is reigned over by the dowager and not the queen. Both houses belong to the heir so there is no worry about the houses keeping up with each other. The head of the family is responsible for them both and what he is doing for them he is doing for them both, his old family and his young one.

The dower house answer to the problem may seem at first sight to be a wealthy man's solution. So it was originally but now the disadvantages of wealth appear to be our peculiar trouble. Today by earlier standards, we are all rich and our difficulties are the difficulties arising from that situation. People who prepare for their own old age could do worse than think along these lines. The actual bricks-and-mortar dower house, specially built for the purpose is, curiously enough, one of the

43 Margery's friend Mary Orr remembered that Margery's mother would regularly say, when staying in D'Arcy House, "Oh I suppose you've put me in the garret again."

better investments today. It is not as if one were constructing something that no one else can live in. A carefully designed container for two people, (which will also accommodate an independent third as and when the need arises), who wish to live a very quiet domestic life with as little housework and as much creature comfort as possible, is not an uncommon requirement for all ages.

If the old establish the dwelling and make the trust and choose the companion then, even so, they should arrange for their heirs to own the fabric even if they themselves retain a life tenancy. They should appoint the family as owners of the house and administrators of the trust, arranging it legally through the solicitor. The psychological and practical effect of this is the difference between the "Smith dower house" and "old Mrs. Smith trying to live near her children". The inclusion of one's own solicitor at this point is important because his natural cautious and sceptical viewpoint prevents one from taking such a step if the heirs' own circumstances do not favour it.

Once in being, the establishment should be as permanent as humanly possible. This is a main ingredient and comes under Protection. The old do not like being moved about or threatened with disturbance of any kind. In any period of development and change all animals prefer quiet and safety. More old people are hurried out of life by being shifted from place to place in well-meaning efforts to help than in any other way.

Life at the dower house proceeds at a different pace and obeys the dictates of a different time of life. Thus if meal-times tend to last very long or to possess a certain Alice in Wonderland inconsequence they are its own meal times and no one else's.

In late middle age a certain amount of to-ing and fro-ing may be most rejuvenating. It also seems part of the whole extraordinary performance. In late life a great many people decide to go back to see either the place of their birth, or the home their ancestors came from. When they first feel they are getting old they often travel miles to do this. It is a natural part of the instinct to take the long view, to see as far as one possibly can. It explains, I think, a mystery which often puzzles the young. They notice that elderly people suddenly give up minding if their ancestors were grand or humble, after perhaps years of telling fairy stories about then. The old simply want to get a clear picture of the sort of people they really were. I now know that this is because before "letting-go" one naturally wishes to understand the long story and observe what one's own particular version of the family type has contributed to it. In a way it is comparable to a trip to the seaside made especially to observe for oneself that a ship really does disappear over the horizon hull first.

In the dower house an uneventful economy is important. Anxieties connected with money do not help the slow process of adaptation and the mutation of one set of strengths into others. The financial arrangements should be definite and the less the old person has to do with any changing details the better. The day-to-day comings-in and goings-out should not now be the old person's affair. The bills and buff envelopes and itinerant collectors must all be someone else's responsibility. These are too much work for anybody whose frontal memory is failing a little and who, in any case, has something else to think about.

The normal tendency today is to persuade old people to try to think about these practical things, which is silly and unkind for few keep up with the changing values of the day and those who do are apt to be made unhappy or afraid by them. The heir is sometimes too grand or too shy to take over what, after all, is the easiest part of his job. He must of course be careful not to take over too soon. Many old people preserve a practical grip on their affairs for a very long time and thoroughly enjoy their participation in these matters. The heir should keep himself alerted to the situation and face the problem resolutely when it arises.

Wherever the money comes from to keep the dower house going – reasonably, it should come from the old people themselves and if so, always, please, through the invaluable solicitor – the heir has to set up what is, in fact, a private, non-profit-making little guest house or nursing home whatever the accommodation may be. The simplest way of arranging the finances is to work out a basic £x per week charge of each old person. All extravagances or economies outside that figure can then be readily recognized. The heir must keep the books, which are vital, and the final say-so must be his or his deputy's. Some of the happiest arrangements of all, emotionally speaking, are those where this method is adopted but the money is made up by the whole family. Each member contributing, as of right, what he feels he wants to and making his own private arrangement with the old person and the administrating heir.

I dwell upon all these details because in many families this is awkward ground. Endless trouble can be caused by members and members-in-law taking a proprietorial interest in the small household. This goes for the most unexpected details, especially of equipment and furnishing. If this endeavour is to succeed it must be kept in mind that the dower house is no doll's house; if new cushions are not kept pristine that cannot be helped. The whole thing is a ritual and a very serious one. Interference must be gently restrained, although help and interest is needed and should be accepted with gratitude. There must be one head of the family (even if he is in partnership with the head of another family) and he must be the payer of bills and orderer of goods, hirer and firer and chooser of advisers; anything less definite than this leads straight to chaos.

The finances of any establishment of this kind are apt to possess a diplomatic quality which would need to be explained to any auditor. Two examples, neither very unusual, may explain what I mean: I knew one elderly lady whose tiny income had been augmented for years by her son until it was sufficient to meet the cost of a very comfortable home with friends.[44] This could only be done by the young man, who was married, if he took advantage of the covenant scheme whereby one person, on making a covenant with another in a lower income group, is permitted by the Inland Revenue to deduct the tax payable at source. The recipient of the gift is then able to claim back the difference between one rate of tax and another — often a considerable amount. In this case the two amounts, the sum actually given and the tax rebate, made up the necessary income for the old lady's maintenance and comfort.

However, she always upset the admittedly complicated arrangement by refusing to understand it. She preferred to believe that she was assisting her son to obtain some sort of tax relief by which he contracted to give her one amount but paid her a lesser one. The twice-yearly sum which was extracted from the Commissioners for her and which was far larger than

44 This was Margery's method of managing her financial support for Em. Letters to the solicitor show her extremely irritated when her mother immediately gave the money away to Grace or to Joyce.

anything she paid in tax, she felt was a little something sent to her by a grateful government because she was such a nice old thing. With this in mind she used to give this "present" away as soon as she got it and it became a regular bi-annual duty of a third member of the family to "borrow" the tax rebate and pay it quietly into the maintenance fund.

In another case an old man, who had a small but adequate pension from his firm, refused point-blank to pay anybody more than six guineas a week for all his requirements, even when they included a night-nurse. He had always saved a pound or so every week for a rainy day and had not noticed that the deluge had arrived. His family met the situation in the time-honoured manner. They discovered that his estate was left to be divided between them and so they borrowed the extra money needed for his maintenance from him and kept careful account. He was delighted to help them out. They paid interest on the loans and he saved that too. When he died the books were produced and any differences in his bequests were adjusted between them.

Incidentally, it was as well that the family made the effort and got him to show them his Will, for it appeared that he was in the habit of keeping it by his bed and correcting it like a proof whenever the idea occurred to him, so by the time it was seen it was not a very legal document. Fortunately he had a solicitor who took the trouble to persuade him to make a new, fair Will which was kept in the solicitor's office while he kept a copy to amend and discuss with the lawyer when he saw him.

The economics of the dower house are peculiar inasmuch as the actual cost seems very often to be met by taking money out of one pocket and putting it into another in what is, virtually, the same suit. It does cost money, of course. Everybody's care and maintenance costs money, but I doubt if expending it in this way is more extravagant than any other and the rewards are infinitely greater. The virtue of the dower house economy is that it usually costs each old person less than he would pay in a private *pension* where there is no nursing; it also has the added advantage that everything that is spent, is spent on the things he happens to want. The pleasures of the dower house when the owners are really happy are tremendous and something that the new children should experience with their parents and grandparents. It is the family plant in being; for a moment complete.

I am aware that in discussing the dower house all the various kinds of inheritance have here become very mixed but that is because they cannot be divided if the situation is to be set out frankly. This is the one time in life when everything a man has he gives away, not only because he no longer needs it but so that he may become unhampered.

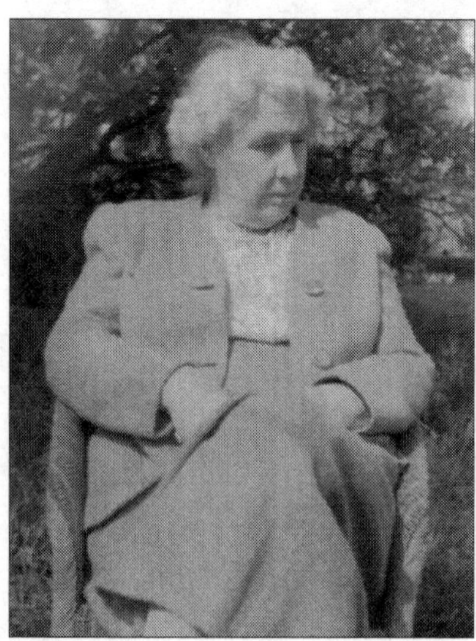

Em Allingham (Hughes) date and place unknown

"So that he may become unhampered"?
Julia Jones

When my mother first moved into Deben View she was constantly putting her possessions out into the corridor. This was often because she didn't recognise that they were hers and also a sincere effort to save trouble for us after she is gone. Some things I picked up and put back in her room, others I stored in case she should ever ask for them again. I was impressed by the unexpected amount of tidying and ordering she had done in the years before she moved. It was correspondingly sad to find previously unknown files of family research torn up and discarded because she had forgotten what they were.

It's one thing Mum deciding for herself to become unhampered: another to have the abilities taken by illness. Now that dementia is advancing, her urge to jettison her possessions seems to have gone, probably because her awareness of things has radically reduced. The things that still matter are those with an emotional extra, with shards of affection clinging nebulously on. The acid-pink teddy bear who shares her sofa is loved for himself and also because she feels that he has come from some of the family's children. She's not at all sure who the children are but frequently asks me to assure them that he is "doing very well".

Margery's dower house sounds Spartan, materially, but contained living reminders of family identity – a sister, a cousin, two daughters/nieces within eyesight across the Square. I have heard Mum talking to a photo of her father late at night, asking him to look after her. We put out pictures of her mother in her wedding dress, on her skis, with her first child; photos of my father and his brother Jack who she also loved. This collection can backfire. "You want me to sleep with all these dead people?" The most successful image is an oil painting of a horse that her mother used to ride. It's highly accomplished, visually clear and is more efficacious than any other single item in helping Mum reorient herself on those dreadful evenings when she is utterly lost in her own surroundings.

Family interpreters are increasingly useful in maintaining the value of Things. Dementia steals the power to recognise, to name, to attribute – but only from the person afflicted. The rest of us can remember that these were Aunt Florence's chairs and we can repeat back Mum's own stories about that long-dead person's affection and generosity. We can tell her that Ros gave her that pretty blouse; Georgeanna the statuette of the foal; Ned sent the postcard, Nick brought the lavish vases of fresh flowers. We know that the givers' names will slip away, along with more technical vocabulary such as "blouse" and "foal", but perhaps she will be helped to remember she is loved. It's good for others to know this too. I sometimes feel I should go round Mum's room sticking labels on her things. Not the labels that may have helped in the earlier stages (TEA TELEPHONE TOILET) nor their pictorial equivalents but chatty little screeds to enable visitors to tell Mum's story back to her – and avert the well-intentioned questions she can no longer answer for herself.

We have to be careful that too much telling doesn't make her feel still more inadequate. We must assure her that she did say thank you, she did write a letter (or I did) and the givers do definitely know that she appreciates her gifts. I repeatedly explain to her about her Alzheimer's and reassure her that other people understand that she really can't remember and this is isn't something she can conquer by trying harder and not being "lazy". I was advised early on that people didn't want to know about their dementia but I haven't found this is true. Telling people not to worry seems likely to make them worry more – especially when they know very well that there's something horribly wrong with their own head. Mum is usually reassured to hear that "there's a lot of it about". I have to bite back my answer to her indignant, "Well someone might have bothered to tell ME!"

One of the legacies my mother will leave with me is a new carefulness at looking at things. Not just her material possessions but the natural world: clouds, leaves, birds, and flowers. This is the opposite of unhamperedness: those clouds that she sees from her sofa are hers, those birds pecking on the patch of grass are her friends. The view from her window is her best possession – except for those very bad days when "they" have been changing it. It would be a dreadful thing to take Mum from "her" view – yet this happens every evening though the winter months. We cannot persuade her to draw the curtains early. Her anxiety is too great. Even yesterday, in April, she commented that "they" had been changing it again – and of course "they" had. The evening light was slanting in from the west to paint the rectangle of lawn a vivid green but the brown fence opposite was in gloomy shadow, the splashes of flower colour muted.

Claudia was away in January and February teaching art on a cruise liner. Reading one of her blog posts aloud to Mum whilst sitting, as usual, on the sofa looking towards the window, gave me a clue what might be happening: "During the last weeks I have taught classes on colour-mixing, perspective, the joys of sketching, the importance of letting the paint dry between washes, and I've impressed on all my students that being an artist, at any level, is a one way ticket from which there is no going back. Even if they never want to take it further, they will from now on see everything around them as colour, shape and line, and their lives will be enriched by the process."[45]

So, if you have lost the specific concepts of "lawn" and "fence", you are seeing the world in abstract terms, whether you choose to or not. You are seeing colour, shape and line and, when the light changes, the relative proportions of the shapes also change. Mum's day-long observations of her view provide more kaleidoscopic permutations than Monet saw in his water-lily pond at Giverny. When evening comes and the shadows lengthen at the dying of the day it's not at all surprising that "spooks" should sometimes creep along that fence as well.

Not that my rationalising helps her very much. I can call this phenomenon "sundowners" and take a surprised interest but she is completely lost and terrified – and therefore, often, very angry. I think it was in early March, not on one of our darkest evenings, when I arrived at Mum's flat at about 5pm to find her standing in the doorway arguing furiously with Eileen, one of the Deben View carers. "I have never had a flat here. I have not been in this terrible place in my entire life."

She saw me and she screamed. Her face was grey and rigid. Then she grabbed me and somehow, from somewhere, summoned sufficient grace to apologise to the carer for startling her. Eileen made some friendly comment and moved off. I walked into the flat with Mum clinging to my arm complaining bitterly that "they" were telling her that she had to sleep in this enormous empty place all on her own and she'd only just arrived here and hadn't seen anyone at all.

45 https://claudiamyatt.co.uk/2016/02/art-lessons-across-the-pacific/

She'd been out with Nick that afternoon so I tried to point to the flowers he'd left her and the map they'd been looking at together on the sofa. She turned to me bitterly. "Do you think that I would have forgotten if my *son* had been here with me?"

There was anger and contempt in her voice but I could hear the panic too. She disengaged herself and began accusing me – I can't remember of what but I knew I was being recast as one of "them". Perhaps she was beginning to have that feeling that she might possibly be mistaken. To have a good row with me would shift the field of battle. I played for time, put the kettle on, asked to use the bathroom. ("Yes – If you think you know where it *is*!") and moved around chatting inanely until I had a tea tray and some biscuits and could lure her to her sofa. She was stiff, angry, rejecting.

I've never been especially good at giving cuddles but for once I managed to do the right thing. I put my arm around her, held her hand and said how hard it must be for her in the evenings and how brave she was to manage it. "I suppose everyone has to," she muttered and turned back into a tired, scared, old lady, crumpling against me, the desperate confusion retreating slightly from her consciousness, perhaps to the edges of our little puddle of physical contact. We sat there partly chatting, partly not, and all the while her free hand was twisting, tugging, pulling at the end of her woollen scarf.

After a while we were able to look together at the water-colour painting of Ramsholt Church that hangs to the side of her sofa. I began to tell her the old story about the day she first arrived in the River Deben with Dad. She'd bought a small yacht (her first) through Dad's newly established agency and he was helping her sail it round to the Deben from the Stour. They stopped at Ramsholt and rowed ashore to the pub. This was

1946 or 1947 and the sale of alcohol was still firmly restricted by the licensing laws. The pub was already closing but "moi toime's me own toime," said the landlord in the rich Suffolk accent that Mum had probably scarcely heard before, fresh as she was from her debutante's flat in Chelsea.

I don't know what he served then, a half of mild-and-bitter probably, but something in the mix of truculence, independence and kindliness established "moi toime's me own toime" as a catchphrase between her and Dad, for ever. Perhaps that moment played some small part of the beginning of the process that would lead to their somewhat unlikely marriage a few years later? Dad's buried in Ramsholt churchyard now and last year my nephew, George, bought her the painting with a sealed bid at a charity auction whilst taking her out for lunch at that same pub.

Parental eyebrows were raised at the scale of George's generosity (he was possibly using his father's cheque book) but the event made a photo for the local paper (another item to stick on her wall) and bought Mum back into relationship with the place where she herself intends to be buried – though not too soon, "I don't want to be dead, Jul." We've since become regulars at their once-a-month communion service, most of which she can neither hear nor understand, but because they use the Book of Common Prayer and the King James Bible, the ingrained rhythms carry her along and well-known phrases surface unexpectedly. "Amen" she says loudly, often a few seconds behind the rest of the congregation. Their hymns are good too, we sing them for hours afterwards and her spiritual experience when she takes communion is intense.

Tunes and stories and scattered phrases are blessed possessions that will not last for ever. It'll be a sad milestone when "moi toime's me own toime" fails to bring the glimmer of a smile. Meanwhile this evening has been salvaged by George's painting and the memories it prompts and her feeling that she is somehow still in a world where there are people who love her. By the time Jane, the bedtime lassie arrives (one of the very best with a twinkle and a hug and words of overt affection), Mum is safely back in her own place and I can return to mine.

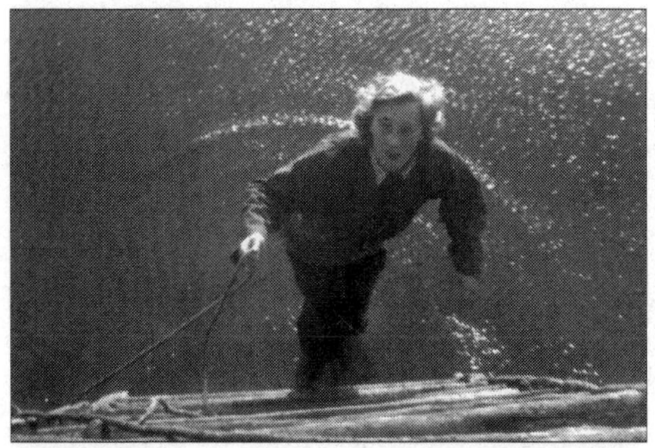

June Scott (later Jones) coming ashore, River Deben c.1947

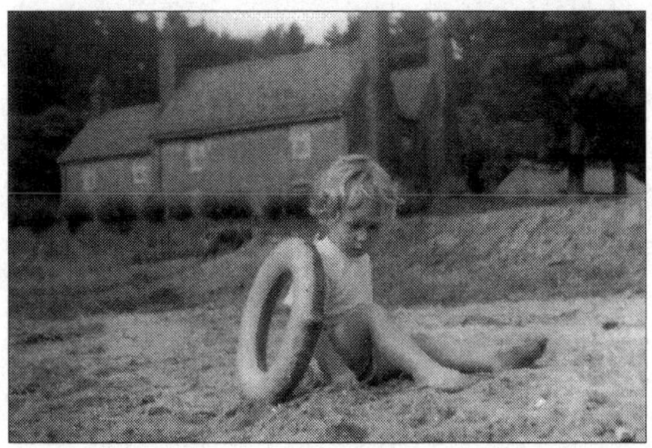

Julia Jones outside the Ramsholt Arms, River Deben 1956

The most delicate of all the dower house requirements
Margery Allingham

The last and most delicate of all the dower house requirements is the Care.[46] In these days it is very difficult to persuade anybody to do any work which he finds unpleasant except by paying him over the odds. In our case that does not arise because the last person to employ is the woman who finds the work so distasteful that she feels it must carry danger or dust money. The Care must be paid well because the one vital thing the job requires is integrity and integrity ill paid is apt to waver. The worst thing a Care can do is to run away. Her salary should be the largest single item in the whole budget but the job should be tailored to fit her and that is where the intelligence, imagination and patience of the heir comes in.

To make this clear perhaps one should consider exactly what one is asking from her. In the first place there is the question of disposition. While it must be admitted that there are people who are a delight to be with in age as in youth, the fact remains that most of us tend to fall into two main groups. There are those who come above the halfway line on the side of the remainder of humanity and those who, quite frankly, do not. At no other time does the difference between the two become so clear as in age. The petals and graces of life are great concealers but in age the hard fruit appears without disguise — "sound and splendid", "good", "sour" or "bitter

46 The word "carer" was not available in this sense at this time.

stuff". Before any heir considers any particular Care for his own old people he should bring himself to face this subject. I doubt if he should confess it to anybody but he should get a very shrewd idea of the facts.[47]

The few saints are the only people who are not exhausting to live with when old. The old are tiring in a very special way, which in itself is misleading, because one seems to associate it almost always with the sadness of what perhaps I may call the prognosis. This angle is liable to obsess us. Few of us care for the idea of everlasting flowers and yet most of us are made sad by the spectacle of a falling bloom. This is so illogical that it must be emotional and can merely mean that we believe that mortal life has many lovely sides. This puts our sadness at the prospect of the failing aged in the same category as our sadness at the sight of the splendid sandcastle doomed as the tide comes in. But that is nostalgic sadness and whatever else it may be it is not exhausting.

That the old are fatiguing can be seen by observing the effects upon the same nurse when working with the old or with the dangerously sick. The former take far more out of her and it does not seem to be the waiting or the putting-up-with, though both are wearying, but appears to be something physical which is as yet imperfectly understood. It has to do with the living force which would seem to flow all the time between people when they are together.[48] It is only interrupted by absence and, curiously enough, by that terrible pride which seems to cut off

47 Elsewhere Margery expands on this thought. "There are those who are charming, thoughtful, sympathetic and even-tempered and it must be admitted that others are demanding, domineering, cantankerous and hypercritical".

48 This idea of a tangible "force" emanating from people or flowing between them was an important concept for Margery and especially in *The Mind Readers* (1965).

the emotional breath. The suppression of this natural flow as in, say, solitary confinement, produces a shocking effect upon the most healthy. The old appear to induce it artificially by having a depleted store of what one can only suppose is the stuff of life itself. At any rate, whatever the cause, the effect produced is remarkably like exhaustion. Those middle-aged people who look after the elderly need more sleep than most and must be revived by contemporary contacts more often than others who do not.

The more comfortable and of consequence one can make the chatelaine the more likely she is to make the extra effort to keep her job and to put up with the little human annoyances which are its greatest disadvantage. Some of her reward comes in "face", and when one finds oneself thinking that it is only a certain kind of woman who lets that worry her it should be recalled that it is just that sort of woman one wants. House-proud women make very good Cares if they are gently persuaded not to let their ruling passion interfere with the comforts of the big room.

The precise duties of the Care vary from family to family but the general principles should not. The newcomer undertakes to provide the old people with the heir's own standard of service but not to replace him. He has his own part to play and indeed she should be restrained should she attempt to usurp it. She must look after the creature comforts of the old people, not as if they were her own but as if she was their own. Moreover, she must put up with exactly what that entails, whatever it happens to be. Any family who asks for more is being unrealistic.

The aspect which is most frequently misunderstood is responsibility. The Care must have integrity but she must not be asked to take responsibility. That is the heir's own affair. If he chooses an unsuitable person that is his fault. He must question cautiously and examine references before engagement on trial and must keep his eyes open until he is completely reassured. He is taking the full liability for another adult and thinking for a life as if it were his own.

The Care should have no hard and fast hours but she should be expected to get out for a while every day and should have a couple of free days to herself every week. This is for health's sake and usually it is more difficult to get her to take them than to keep to them.

The wages of a geriatric attendant in one's own part of the country are an indication of the sum a Care would ask.[49] A dower house Care is a good job for both men and women. A technically unskilled person is only asked to do the kind of work at which thousands of widows and grass widows up and down the country are very good indeed. She is merely required to run a tiny labour-saving house, exactly as if it were her own proud possession, economically on a budget but without interference unless the result proves unsatisfactory. She must shop and cook light meals in a model kitchenette and clean and home-wash all but large items in a machine. In fact, in all these respects she should behave like a valued landlady of that Victorian kind patronised by Sherlock Holmes and Dr Watson. Her job is to do all she can to help and make happy two old "star" boarders and to keep a daughterly eye upon them, but after that her responsibility ends.

In cases of emergency she must telephone the heir for instructions as well as cope to the best of her ability until

49 Margery was offering "£1 a day and all found. Then, after six months satisfactory service, £100 a year in an annuity so she has something to retire on."

appropriate help arrives, but she must not be left with trouble which she cannot manage. The degree of emergency which merits a call is one of those important points which must be decided between heir and Care. It is bound to vary in almost every case. When the heir is a woman she may want to be called on slighter pretexts than a man but in every case it is a matter for adjustment. Old people, like young ones, often amuse themselves by playing up one person against another and some revel in dramatic display, so that for the first week or so the emergency rate may be alarmingly high. The old do not settle quickly and their rattled nerves can produce all sorts of upsets, from stomach trouble to fits of rage and tears. It is part of the late fireworks of life and is nearly always a passing phase. A good Care who is anxious to settle herself can often soothe these much better than the family, but she must be backed up if necessary.

Mobile old people who retain their legs longer than their heads can provide some alarming moments. I remember one Care telephoning a family at ten o'clock at night to say: "Your Aunt has climbed out of the kitchen window and has been brought back by a motorist who says she has asked him to drive her to London. She is being absolutely charming and I'm afraid he believes her and not me. What shall I do?"[50] That is the time for professional interference but it should be recalled that senility and delirium or the delusions of uraemia are all very different conditions even if the symptoms do appear the sane. That particular aunt recovered for quite a while after that incident but everyone was very lucky to have a sensible Care.

Now that there are so many schemes for training, a Dower House Care Service could be sponsored by an

50 Anecdote refers to Grace Russell.

organisation drawing its raw material from that large group of older housewives who, perhaps, have never worked outside their homes before. When they come to do so, they should remember that the dower house Care is not a nurse, nor yet a companion, although she may serve as both on occasions. She is certainly not a domestic but she must not mind if either of her "boarders" assume she is one: no one else must. She is the heir's "forty-second cousin" and if the old people sack her twice a day in the first week she must wait for him before even noticing it.

There are dangers here as there are in all human relationships. Many people are highly responsible and enjoy assuming authority but, simple though this can make things for the heir, it should never be encouraged. The Care should never handle money save the house-keeping and that should be accounted for as it would be in many private households. The "kitchen book", that invaluable ledger, is very well understood these days. The Care should never be consulted as to the economics of the whole concern. She may seem like a partner but she is not one and she must never on any account have any financial understandings or promised legacy arrangements with her boarders. In any question of this sort the old people must be persuaded to consult their solicitor whose professional skill will guide him how to deal with any situation which may arise.

The Care has her own quarters where – in some cases where the house is large enough – she could keep a school child. She has her own street door, her own dignity as the mistress of a fine little establishment, and all she has to do is to see that the people in her big front room are so happy that they do not want any change. She is well paid and she can save it almost all for her own retirement. If there is any trouble or disaster she has an authority to turn to instantly who is guaranteed to do something at once.

It sounds almost too good to be true and it is – if one is assuming that the few negative items mentioned above are in any way negligible, or if one overlooks the one important thing. The item the dower house Care is expected to give is her life, however much comfort one is able to give her. She is asked to make the dower house a home, which means that though she may not always be there, she is thinking of it all the time. No one who will not do this is any good. Mercifully, a great many women will and will enjoy it and make a "go" of it.

Perhaps one should pause here to hint at the sort of criticism a head of the house may earn if he establishes a dower house: "I wish I had £x a week and all found for lying on my bed and looking at telly all day!" "There was dust under auntie's bed." "Her place looks all right but theirs is squalid!" "Can't she make Auntie stop wearing that awful old cardigan?" "I don't think Mrs Thing ought to have that child/visitor/local gossip in her sitting room."

There may be complaints from the old people themselves. "I dropped my book and called and called." "She was out for quite half an hour!" "I told her I like to keep my medicine here. Sometimes I forget and take it twice but it's my inside!"

The Care is unlikely to be any less human and fallible than anybody else: "I don't know if I ought to tell you but, when they are alone, they criticise *you*." "Mrs Ass tells me that if I owned this house myself and was letting the room I should make a fortune." "Your aunt slapped me! I didn't tell you because we're all so happy here but I did mention it to Mrs Ass." Any of these remarks can be the forerunner of the kind of crisis one gets in the soap operas and they are the stuff of home life. This is the

inheritance which is the heir's own and ought not to be missed if his own old age is not to find him an apprehensive tyro when the time comes.

In these days of Government health and packaged cures for most things there is a great danger of young people thinking of old age as a mortal illness, which is, of course, not the true picture at all. There is no disease in a death from old age although an illness is often contracted during the last days of life. The term nursing has changed in meaning, too, and tends nowadays to make one think either of brain operations or having-an-affair-with-a-doctor, according to which school of television programme one favours.[51] The presence of the old in one's immediate circle, however, does mean that an elementary knowledge of the care of a human body which is not as new as it was is a useful thing. This is not sick nursing but rather the ordinary adult information that one collects on one's journey through life and is comparable with that knowledge of mechanics which can be gained from driving the same car for a very long time.

As far as general health is concerned the main difference between the old and the young is that the old are more susceptible to the bad effects of change, cold and virus infection. They are more liable to suffer from night cramps and stiffness of joints and muscles than the young. However, by that time most or their pet illnesses and cures will be known to them and to their doctor. The fears in the back of most people's minds in connection with the later stages of life are the old wives' whispers and nurse-y mutterings about incontinence and bed sores. The young, who are naturally fastidious, are, I think, properly horrified and determinedly ignorant.

51 For example the popular ITV soap opera *Emergency Ward 10* which ran from 1957-1967.

However, nothing is as fearful as fear itself and when one has cornered one's nurse (for this is no subject for the doctors) and sorted out the facts from the drama, the problems of both are not as dreadful as they first appear. They are both undignified and that is the worst thing about them. Since neither is likely to occur for some time to come and then mercifully only for a short while, they are hardly matters on which to expend a lifetime of dread. The first thing to remember is that neither may occur.

There is nothing very mysterious about bed sores. I think I can best explain to the non-technical mind by saying that in healthy old age one dies like an apple does. You must turn it over and over, since in time its own weight will bruise it. Preservation of the skin at all points where the main weight is carried, not forgetting the head and the heels, is most important.

At this time of life the visits of the nurse are more important than the doctor's. If there is incontinence she must have a rubber underlay, old sheets and rolls of that cellulose paper which have taken much of the drudgery out of this kind of nursing. Nurse will have her own preferences as to what is needed and know the best methods to be employed. Nowadays the visiting auxiliary, backed up by a State Registered nurse for more skilled attentions, can both be approached through the doctor and National Health Service. To the average family they are invaluable because they are knowledgeable and responsible.

All the same, the actual moving of a very old person who is no light weight can prove not only exhausting but well-nigh impossible for the amateur. It can also be very uncomfortable for the old person. In recent years a remarkable answer to this worry has appeared called a "Talley bed". This is a mattress, a corrugated alternating air bed which is worked by

a very small amount of electricity and which shifts the pressure automatically. It is imperceptible and the sleeper is unaware of the very slight and gradual movement. Aunt had no troubles of this kind in the last weeks of her life any more than her mother had done, but the one case took the strength out of two youngish women whereas the other was no physical strain on anybody. This device was called an "Alternating Pressure Point Pad unit" and we hired it from the Talley Surgical Instrument Company of London.

All these nursing details belong to a much later stage than most of the rest of this book. Granny lived with me for close on nine and a half years after she was ninety before I heard about pressure points. Our problems before then were much more of the "tired-ordinary-self" variety; forgetfulness, finding it more and more difficult to read, however strong the glasses, and finally the sad day when, despite the hearing aid, the BBC announcers began to mumble.

The strong and determined old person whose legs have become unreliable can wreck a house by finding hand grips where none was intended and can hurt himself badly as the moulding round doors comes away or a washbasin used as a pull-up is torn bodily from the wall. Fortunately, this sort of trouble has occurred before – although, I believe, most old people and their children are taken by surprise by it – and there are many devices which are well worth tracking down at any of the big medical supply stores. These firms are listed in the Yellow Pages and between them they can produce something to meet practically every problem imaginable. It is worthwhile approaching them when faced with a difficulty which a mechanical aid might alleviate.

Take them the problem and let them suggest an answer.

When you have it, take up the question with the National Health. The State, having shouldered the expense of sickness, is dickering with the expense of old age and in the end will shoulder that too. Meanwhile it is up to those most concerned to help it towards efficiency by finding out what it can do if we take advantage of the services it already provides. It is an almost free service on a par with the upkeep of roads. If it can allow the device it will. Even rubber mattresses and cot beds can all be lent free on a householder's signature. Other expendable items are obtainable on prescription in the usual way. When considering expense it is as well to remember that many people who could claim a supplementary pension do not do so because they are either too proud or too frightened of the possible red tape this would involve. Many of them do not want the trouble of dealing with "the Government". Bureaucracy with its forms and queries is often intimidating and a certain time-waster when one has other things to think about and time is getting short. It is up to the heir to look into this side of his old people's affairs.

The cot bed is needed for a curious aberration which sometimes afflicts the very old late in the day. Suddenly, they take a delight in sliding out on to the ground with the object of making one put them back again. This can appal one if it is unexpected and becomes a bore when it is. The answer is an ordinary child's cot but of larger dimensions. There is also a valuable chrome steel object for pulling oneself up in the bath. This fastens round the base of the taps and is a great help when used with a non-slip mat placed in the bottom of the bath. There is also a device to make tap-turning easier.

The most useful contraption which we built ourselves was a crash barrier set three feet from either bed. We made the beds high, so that the floor beneath them could be easily swept, and we made them fixtures. There are people who would not like a cubicle with curtains although ours was made of two single four-poster beds and looked most imposing. In this case two small open bedrooms can be made with expanding walls in the same space. The important thing is that the temperature between bedroom and sitting room should be the same and that a person in bed should not be necessarily cut off from what is going on in the main room. When one is merely "retired" the cottage can be used in the normal way but when one is old there is not quite the same sharp division between being up and being in bed as there is in one's middle years. It is sometimes pleasant to potter about all day getting up or going to bed.

Perhaps I should explain that all our old people were very heavy folk and very independent inasmuch as they disliked fuss or assistance. However, one of the most usual annoyances in old age is to find oneself giddy on first getting out of bed. We found that a variety of mishaps could occur in these circumstances and we overcame them by taking the following precautions:Between the beds, set three feet from each, we erected our barrier. This was a two-barred fence, very like those which are set before the gates of primary schools. It was shaped like a radiator towel-rail but was a little longer and it was made of two-inch zinc piping with rounded angles. This was let down twelve inches into the concrete below the floor. It had a flat circular collar to each foot to keep it steady. It sounds hideous but it was enamelled and it proved the most valuable ally we had. Its great virtue was that it was almost more solid than anything else in the building. It could be used when dressing, as ballet dancers use the bar; a wheeled chair could be moored against it safely and one could pull oneself up by it and be absolutely certain that it would never even tremble. It was also used to carry blankets and clothes and it made a permanent demarcation between the two bedroom spaces in the one curtained cubicle. When the time came to remove it, it unscrewed and the holes in the concrete were filled up and the floorboards plugged.

Another useful aid was a walking machine which helped to keep Aunt Maud exercised, happy and straight. Holding oneself bent and forcing one's organs slightly out of place is a bad consequence of any disability which affects only one side. A bicycle basket fitted on the front of the machine will add to the independence of the user as also would the wearing of an apron with large pockets, but these details should be left to the wishes of the old.

In our experience we had observed people who, when dealing with the problems of others, cannot help trying to do then some sort of moral good at the same time – on the side, as it were, "with the left hand in passing". We were all adamant that no attempt to steer our old ladies must be made by us that was not absolutely vital to their physical well-being. It was to be the converse of the nursery, not a repetition of it.

In practice this resolved itself into an honest attempt, within the limits of sanity, to give them nothing they did not want and everything they wanted, the moment they wanted it. They had all lived for over seventy years trying to get just this. Their souls were their own and it seemed to us that the remaining few years of their lives were still very much their own affair of which we were but a junior part. We had not to instruct them, they were to instruct us about ourselves and what we learned from them was our chief inheritance.

I fear the obstinate moralists must be very clear-thinking

indeed if they are to follow this. For their guidance I would point out that we were not just looking after any old people. They were our old people with whom we were running in the Relay.

Since the National Health is a service and not human, the thing it does not do is to come and hunt you up. It is not the doctor's private charity nor yet the Government in disguise but a very complex well-thought-out machine we have all bought between us. It takes a little exploratory work before one gets the hang of how to use it to its best advantage. What the State cannot supply at home is all the care and all the administration and all the thought. It will be a pity if it ever does because the real home that people live and die for and remember for ever, is not the pretty room, nor the home-made cake but the idiotic incident, the laugh, the idiosyncrasy, authority romping, mother playing the goat, the instalment of one's own story, which could belong to no one else, caught in time for always.

When Granny was first kept in bed she frightened me one morning with a story of two great black birds which had appeared in her room and stolen her bread and butter. I assumed that her mind was going at last and the type of delusion struck me as terrible, although she seemed singularly undisturbed by it. When I went up again sometime later she was lying asleep with one arm on the coverlet and on the long sleeve of her white calico nightdress I saw, to my amazement, three large broad arrows in soot. I looked round and saw them everywhere, all over the pillows and the white cloth on the bedside table. Convict 99 could not have been more firmly stencilled. We found the egg spoon in the fireplace and the chatter of the jackdaws in the chimney explained the mystery. It was quiet, I suppose, and she was a very gentle, welcoming old lady.

"A very gentle, welcoming old lady"?
Julia Jones

Margery's love for her Granny is one of the most appealing features of *The Relay*. The anecdote of Emily Jane's sweet thanks when Margery and Joyce were turning her in bed stayed with me from my first reading back in the 1980s when elder care wasn't even a smudge on my horizon. Later, as my mother's equilibrium declined, I became afraid that she would never exhibit the same grace. Attempts to persuade her to accept help when she was still living in her cottage had all failed and people's feelings were hurt. I imagined that I would be spending the foreseeable future smoothing over outbursts and pleading with people to stay. There was a bizarre incident early in her tenancy at Deben View when she described to me in dramatic detail how she had shouted at and sacked the supplementary carer we were then employing. It was something inexplicable to do with the carer touching some precious glasses that Mum was keeping safe for Nick. She told me exactly where they had been standing – in the corridor outside her flat – and what she'd said and how the carer's expression had changed, how deflated she had been and how she'd left without a word.

I was horrified of course. I already suspected that the person in question might be quite vulnerable beneath her highly competent manner, and I wondered frantically how I could minimise the damage from this semi-public humiliation. I settled in the end on a carefully-worded, hand-delivered letter of appreciation and apology. The carer was astounded.

As far as she was aware, the incident had never happened. She had called at Mum's flat as usual. The visit had felt perfectly normal, though she had thought perhaps Mum was a little "vague". There had been no scene in the corridor, no hard words, no accusations, no sackings. Not in her perception. But no matter how fast I back-pedalled she was then so alarmed by Mum's capacity for delusion that she resigned anyway.

Margery once described her mother, Em, as being "not really safe with people" and that too has stayed among my selection of comforting phrases. Margery has sometimes felt like an unknown big sister and I am strengthened by the perceptions and expressions that she has unwittingly passed on. I realise, however, that this isn't necessarily personal, it's what a good writer achieves. I wish Margery had written even more about the delicacy of relationships between the family member, professional or semi-professional care-worker in this section of *The Relay* rather than moving on to the practical aspects of protection and physical care.

It's an interesting reflection of priorities, however, fifty years ago. Margery was used to employing people within her household and was confident establishing job expectations and the boundaries of responsibility. From 1931, when she and Pip moved out of London, they had always been living in a mixed household where some people were employers, some employed and others (such as her pre-war amateur housekeeper Cooee) occupied the potentially difficult middle ground between friend and employee. There had been "set-outs" in those early days but by the late 1950s such uncertainties were generally past.

The NHS, however, was still quite new and she was clearly fascinated by its potential. Today most UK families may be able to take the availability of handrails and continence aids more easily for granted; establishing ways of working in personal partnership with medical professionals and employed care-workers may feel significantly harder. Margery was unperturbed by the currently divided paths of health and social care: some aspects free, others means-tested, services very often appearing unable to communicate with one another despite individual good intentions. "The State, having shouldered the expense of sickness, is dickering with the expense of old age and in the end will shoulder that too," she wrote cheerfully. "Meanwhile it is up to those most concerned to help it towards efficiency by finding out what it can do if we take advantage of the services it already provides."

She had cared for Emily Jane from the early 1940s with very little State assistance. This new 1960s world of free health care felt encouraging. "It takes a little exploratory work before one gets the hang of how to use it to its best advantage. What the State cannot supply at home is all the care and all the administration and all the thought." Her final sentence is still true.

Margery identified Protection, Companionship and Care as the human requirements for a contented old age – and that's what her dower house scheme was able toprovide. In our situation, safe purpose-built facilities, basic personal care and some general oversight comes with the extra care housing but the element of companionship has proved more difficult. Mum was a solitary person even in marriage and remained so for most of her thirty-plus years of widowhood. Certainly not "a gregarious old jolly bird anxious to chirp her last in concert," to quote *The Relay*. My brothers and I will gladly supply "all the administration and all the thought" but, as Mum's illness has eroded her capacity for both practical and emotional independence, we have discovered that our family resources are not sufficient for companionship. Our own version of the "forty-second cousin" is not a full-time, live-in carer but the discreetly paid friend or specialist support worker, calling at pre-arranged times and building up their own relationships of trust and friendship.

This is not always without difficulty. The phrase "living with" dementia seems to recognise the presence of that additional, unpredictable third party – as the first carer and I so unexpectedly discovered. Since then my forty-second cousins and I have got better at adopting a team approach, though the wild card of mum's brain fizz still regularly double-crosses us. Some of us are good at walking, some read poetry, others sing songs or look at photographs: we all do our best to communicate with one another and try to analyse problems. Other friends and family members are involved in their various ways and I have learned to refer to myself as the "primary carer".

That's helpful to Mum, I hope. She needs a single focal point. I suppose that was what happened on DD-day, I drunk to the bottom of my pewter mug and discovered the King's Shilling twinkling there. Perhaps if Ned's well-meaning friend had told me I was going on a "voyage" with Mum – not that clichéd journey – I might have responded more graciously. You can recruit a crew if you're off on a voyage; you can organise a watch-system.

It wasn't until Nicci and I set out on John's Campaign in November 2014 that I regularly began describing myself as a carer rather than a daughter. Margery's word "heir" won't do. It is, as she says, ruined by its association with material inheritance – although, somehow, we need to hold on to her insistence that there is a prospect of gain as well as loss in this altered relationship. The word carer wasn't available in its modern sense when Margery wrote *The Relay* and although it might have helped her in her indecision between the "Care" and the "Chatelaine" for her paid worker, it isn't especially helpful as a designation for the loving volunteer.

There are care-givers and care-workers and in my innocence I made an assumption that the c-word was derived from some root in a Romance language. I warmed myself into my new role with the preciousness of the Italian *cara*, the tenderness in the Welsh *cariad*: affection mingled with solicitude. That seemed about right. One can always feel a little better about being an "amateur" rather than a professional if you allow the word to remind you that you are doing whatever it is for love *(amo, amas,amat…)*. Unfortunately, I discover that "carer" in its current sense comes from Old English *cearu* – woe, distress etc. Perhaps this is a recognition of the imminence of what Margery calls "the Prognosis", or perhaps because caring has been experienced by too many people as a lonely, exhausting and essentially negative experience. At the same time as Margery was contemplating *The Relay*, the Rev Mary Webster was picking up her pen to write the letter to *The Times* that sparked the Carers Movement. She wished to join with others in order to combat her feelings of personal isolation and social invisibility.

Cearu indeed. Despite the successes of the Carers Movement, despite the many reports and White Papers on Social Care, there are still many hundreds of thousands of people, frequently elderly themselves, taking responsibility entirely alone, without the support of wider family, forty-second cousins or even the essential "care-workers".[52] I recently completed a questionnaire for a final year university student

52 *Caring into Later Life*, a joint report from Carers UK and Age UK, states that 87,000 people aged over 85 are carers, either for their partners or for aging disabled children. This figure has risen by 128% over the last 10 years.

in which every question seemed to assume that I would be suffering health problems and a sense of worthlessness. I don't. I often feel stressed and anxious, as one does when undertaking any major responsibility. I feel ignorant and inadequate, often guilty, frequently emotional. But I'm not the lonely martyr that the questions appeared to expect.

It wasn't until I reached the end of the survey, feeling thoroughly fraudulent and wishing I'd never called myself a carer, that I realised where the design fault lay – at no point had I been asked how much of the care I provided directly myself, hands-on. Yes, I am Mum's "principal carer". Yes, I take responsibility for her overall well-being as best I can. Yes, she is somewhere in my mind almost every hour of the day (and that's perhaps why imaginative writing feels so peculiarly impossible) but I would have no life of my own at all if it were not for existence of the Deben View "lassies".

Deben View is run by a housing association in partnership with social services. When Mum moved in she was presented a list of names, qualifications and job titles of the people who would be implementing her agreed "care plan". She took a look and decided it was quite impossible that she should remember so many names so she began to call them her "lassies". I hoped fervently that this would be understood, as intended, as a friendly designation. It wasn't only that Mum's previous responses to paid care had ended badly, I worried also that, because she had been brought up as a rich man's daughter in a house run by staff, she might revert in some way to a snobbish, class-based behaviour.

I was completely wrong. Firstly, she had been brought up to acknowledge professionalism. Clearly it would have been unthinkable in her childhood home to behave otherwise than with extreme respect towards Nellie the housemaid, Carter the groom or "Goggy" (Mrs Ovenden) the cook. I have also come to suspect that Mum, as a child, was not confident in her own value or her parents' love. The kindness she received in her earliest years – from Goggy in particular – has left her with a lifelong debt of gratitude. I discover that she is hugely responsive to kindness. I don't think I knew this before. Morning after morning now when Francis or I ring her up, she says, "Oh I've such a lovely time with lassie!" And she *does* say thank you.

It is not uncomplicated. The dementia nurse told me how crucial the first five years of life are to the way many people with dementia behave as the illness progresses. Too late to change that. Mum's nanny preferred her talented and charming older brother – or so Mum believes. She loved her brother too and regularly mentions his cleverness, kindness, poshness, general superiority. Theirs was a very Alpha-male household and Mum is left with a tangled mass of resentments, loyalties and inferiorities to deal with, as well as her love, gratitude and intense nostalgia. I may be wrong to single out the nanny but there is something that makes her very quick to rebel against those she perceives to be in positions of power. While she loves her "lassies", she can be shockingly rude and angry towards their seniors. Through this deconstructive process of dementia I feel I am seeing further back into my mother's life than I have ever done before. It explains, of course, various aspects of my own upbringing – and therefore aspects of me.

Despite dementia, Mum is clever. This is touching and painful to observe. On the emotional level where she functions now she is responsive and sensitive – and can be unreasonably offended. Her's is the nervous sensitivity of a very young child with the dignity of a senior citizen. She does not trust indiscriminately – it is *her* lassies to whom she is grateful, not any stranger sent along by an agency, charming though they may individually be. This is some sort of indefinable, emotional knowing, even without explicit recognition. I can frequently guess which carer has been there in the morning by the songs that Mum is singing. If it's been "best lassie" I'll be treated to "Mademoiselle from Armentieres" or "Three old ladies locked in a lavatory" which Mum finds wickedly hilarious. "She's a real pal, that one," says Mum, "I really must try to remember her name."

I too wish I could name all the "dear lassies" who leaven the first half hour of showering, dressing, pill-administration and toast-making with a song, a little dance and expressions of affection. I am grateful to Deben View for amending their routes so that Mum gets the same carer visiting at breakfast and lunchtimes and then (crucially) the same person at teatime and bedtime. The difference that it makes to me, when I leave her in the evening, to be able to say definitely that Jane/Alice/Kim/Shareen/Beth/Naomi/Sally will be here in half an hour to help you to bed, is huge.[53] Trust is surely something that one reposes in a known human being. And it's not only my mother who needs this, it's everyone who is living with dementia and whose care is shared with others. To assume that because someone can no longer remember names they cannot discriminate between people is breathtakingly crass.

Partnership-building between families and institutions, even non-institutional institutions like extra care housing, can be surprisingly difficult. It is as if no one quite accepts that overall responsibility can be shared – indeed must be shared. Caring alone for a person with dementia isn't good for that

53 Julie/Cheryl/Shona/Rosie /Sandra/Katherine/Leanne/Vickie/Nicky/Eileen – thank you too. And the team leaders and the night staff who I never see.

person themselves. I notice Mum getting faintly bored when it's only me she sees all day. Complete dependency is also highly risky. Unsupported family carers become exhausted, they break down. Yet the moment the cared-for person enters some other form of living it may feel as if the cut-off from the family is final: that it's the parting at the workhouse gate. "I asked the wee daughter why she was so upset," said a senior Scottish nurse who had been the manager of a residential home, "an' she told me that she'd always bought her mam a fish supper on her way home from work on a Friday. It had been a highlight of their week an' she couldna bear to think she'd no be doing it anymore. So I said to her 'Why do you think that your mam'll no be wanting her fish supper on a Friday? This is her home. You'll bring it to her here.'"

Families feel guilt and betrayal. Professionals are too quick to assume that families have given up completely because they have given up something. It was hard to persuade the carers at Deben View that they didn't have to manage Mum's rages and distress all by themselves. She is still my mother and I will still try to help her and in many ways I have the best chance of doing so. Recently I was talking to Adrienne, the team leader who had lured Mum to the telephone on the evening of our epic row. She hadn't actually heard the moment when I had screeched at Mum to "go away and die you silly cow" and I thought she looked shocked when I told her. Then she laughed and said, "Well I had no more trouble after that. Your mother went to bed like a lamb and slept all night."

We were in a meeting with the dementia specialist. She asked me whether my mother and I had often had rows. "Mmm, yes, possibly…" "Perhaps that made it a safe way for her to get rid of her own anger and frustration?" she suggested.

Maybe... There are certainly times when I can see that Mum is wanting to pick a fight. She's always been emotionally more nimble than I am and now that she genuinely can't remember what she said thirty seconds earlier it makes her quicker still. I have noticed an expression of glee when she has provoked me into yelling at her to tell her to stop yelling at other people.

It's not a good strategy though. I hate having rows with Mum just as much or even more than I ever did. They make me feel inadequate and clod-hopping and resentful and emotionally exhausted. Arguing with a person with dementia is perhaps not unlike arguing with a toddler. It's a no-win. You need a quick diversion strategy or you need to leave the room. And you are not arguing with a toddler, you are arguing with someone who is older than yourself, has seen more of life than you have and who is ill. It isn't a right thing to do.

When Mum was upset last week the bedtime lassie brought her to the phone and helped her make a call. I'd been there at teatime so I knew who was on duty. "Your mother's not sure where she is," she said. "She wants you to tell her whether it's safe." "Hello, Mum. Yes I do know exactly where you are. You're in your room at Deben View and I'll be down to see you in the morning. I know the person who you're with as well. Her name is Alice." "Hey, lassie, is your name Alice?" "Yes, I'm Alice." "She says her name is Alice." "Yes, she's Alice and I know her and I like her very much." "Hey, lassie, she says she likes you. What's your name?" "I'm Alice." "She says she's called Alice." "Yes, that's right, it's Alice, Mum. You're okay with her. Sleep well now and I'll see you in the morning."

That's how shared care is meant to work, I think. So no-one is loaded beyond their capacity to bear, including the old person who most needs our help.

Old people tend to try and save their steps
Margery Allingham

Old people tend to try and save their steps by loading themselves in a way which would unnerve a Chinese juggler ("I've brought my tray, your dressing gown, pussy and the long cobweb brush…") and very few of them heed any admonitions on the subject because next time they contemplate going downstairs they think all over again what a nuisance it was to come up and how they had better collect all they may need and take it down NOW. It really is quicker and safer in the long run to have no stairs or steps anywhere near them.

No one under the age of forty-five ought to have any idea how important the single level requirement is and after that age it should be only a suspicion. There comes a time when it is all the difference between smooth water and a choppy sea. In my experience old people fall over almost anything. There are a few well padded, solid-boned old bodies who can roll about like babies with remarkably little ill effect but they are rare. Far too many old bones snap like twigs and the shock and pain of the experience can be the beginning of serious trouble. It is disquieting to recall that more bones are broken by falls in the house than are caused by accidents on the roads.

Other safeguards should include outside doors which lock and have notices on them requesting callers to go slow. Those jolly electric meter readers, bakers and delivery men who rush in like visiting express trains, can have a shocking effect on someone whose whole habitation is becoming rather ramshackle. Boisterousness is seldom appreciated and this includes the cavorting of children.

Many people just before the point of "let-go" begin to hoard for the future as if for a siege. The explanation is the old one: "I'd better buy a dozen toothbrushes NOW while I remember so that I don't have to come all this way to the shops again". Anyone who has had much to do with the old will recognize this problem of impedimenta. There may be drawers full of clothes which no longer fit or unopened parcels from unlikely shops. Army Surplus stores seem a great favourite. Some old people hoard bottles of medicine which go bad or woollens which tend to collect moth but are greatly prized. The ideal storage space should be visible but not very accessible so that the goods can remain obviously safe without encouraging constant examination.

The dower house is an anteroom; in it some temperaments wait lazily as if they were thinking of rousing themselves to go to a lovely bed; some fidget as if they were hanging about on a railway station; and some as if they were in a dentist's waiting room.

In the unregenerate twenties "old ladies' bedrooms" was a term of opprobrium for any kind of oppressive atmosphere and it is worth recalling it. The truth of the matter is that any nose becomes acclimatised even if the owner is practically suffocated. It is up to the young who are moving in and out and, of course, to the Care, to keep an eye on the ventilation. Those sprays which allegedly kill odours are not advised. It is real new air which is needed, not the synthetic kind.

Light is a matter of taste. Some old people like a very bright light but some hate it and, as they are not always quite sure what it is that is irritating them, it is as well to explore this preference; it is very seldom a thing which changes from day to day. Heating too, is a matter of choice. The only important things about it are that it must be adequate and must be reliable. It should be as simple as possible. If one has the open fire which the old people of a generation ago loved so much, then it should be fitted with a back-boiler and a couple of radiators to prevent all the heat from being in one place and it must have a strong guard.

Most old people resent this precaution but better a battle of persuasion than the ghastly accidents which can and do so often occur. If gas is used then it should be fitted with one of the safety devices which light the gas the moment it is turned on. A naked flame should never be without a guard. Electric cords, too, are sources of trouble and should never be long enough to trail. It is no good relying upon anyone to watch these. They must be bad-memory-proof and the electric convector and oil-filled radiator are safest of all.

Furniture is not quite as simple as one might suppose. For old people the furniture should be divided into the heavy kind which not only is not meant to move but is seen to be immovable, and the very lightly sort which runs smoothly on large ball-castors or wheels. In the dower house quarters all door-furniture should be kept overhauled. Screws slip out of handles and plastic fittings splinter very easily. Solid steel grips as hand-holds can be placed at strategic points to fit needs which become apparent. A chromium steel contrivance to provide arms can be obtained for the lavatory but it must be rigid. Nothing is more useless than a safety gadget which is unsteady. If one is building, then it is worth while putting in a wide old-fashioned lavatory seat over the modern pan. These can be made with arms and are very fashionable, I notice, among the connoisseurs of gracious living.

That is how the dower house idea works out in modern times and it may be criticised by those who see it as a method whereby one pays a staff and does the hardest part of the work oneself but that, as I have been repeating all through this book, is the object of the whole procedure. The dower house permits the family, by uniting its strength into a bundle of sticks, to afford their old people the care and protection which it is its privilege to supply and their right to accept.

Some older people who prefer to put their trust primarily in capital may sometimes find themselves saving up for old age as if it were some sort of unpleasant holiday – full of bad weather, sickness and crooked landladies. It proves to be much more of a job than this when it comes; much more of a development. Young people can easily observe this for themselves if the old people in question are not the blank-faced strangers of the first-class carriage but those known and loved.

The principles of the dower house can be applied to almost any sort of establishment which can be modified to fit the essential requirements. If one were rich enough, I do not see why they could not be obtained in an hotel and one would certainly achieve them in the space occupied by one and a half Council flats for old people.

Local government attempts at housing the old have made many leaps forward; the Warden system usually works well, especially when it is linked with those small units that provide some communal amenities. In other designs, more suitable for young marrieds than the elderly, the old find themselves before the moment of "let-go" with no heir and no protector. They get into all sorts of muddles and are very difficult to help.

After the "let-go", sooner or later, they have to become the occupiers of scarce hospital beds which they neither need nor like and which cost the State an enormous amount of money. In hospital certain disciplines and confiscations have to be instigated and so the State becomes the heir in spite of itself and naturally inherits nothing but abuse.

This is all very well when there are no rightful heirs or when families are going to the bad and giving up the Relay. The State's answer is very much better than no care at this time. Far too often this version of the story leaves the good family, which has insufficient money to compete with the often rather extravagant State in the matter of physical amenities, being squeezed out of the Relay. This really must not be allowed to happen because if the community takes away a man's responsibility to his forefathers, the community is depriving his son of his physical, mental and emotional inheritance, and that is too much control altogether. We must not become a nation of broilers even if our gay little ticky-tacky nesting boxes are beginning to suggest that idea too vividly for comfort.

I should have thought that a wise local government (whose pidgin all this is) would be able to devise some scheme to meet this problem and could evolve a system of letting the old people's dwellings to their families, off-setting some of the cost by rates relief or other like grants, but saving itself thereby a lot of money on hospital maintenance. This would bolster the family's responsibility in the matter instead of undermining it. Young people often gang up to provide play schools for their youngest. There is no reason at all why they should not do as much for their eldest.

A large communal dower house would be impractical because the administration would be impossible unless the basic idea was sacrificed. Each new housing estate could include a few labour-saving bungalows or flats designed for "Two and the Care". These could be let on short leases, as they were needed, to an heir or to a partnership of two responsible house-holding heirs who would then make their own arrangements. It would require intelligent invention in the first place and most wise administration because there is Care to consider, but we have some fine local administrators of this kind in Britain.

More expensively, a commercial undertaking could make a modest profit by building and letting a series of detached or semi-detached cottages in the grounds of a Guest house or Club where the younger people could stay, or at least eat, when visiting. This would turn out to be a new version of the present Old People's Home but with a highly important difference. Here there would have to be one professional residential Deputy on the spot at the main house who would act directly for each heir and be paid by him and would employ the Care. The young people would rent the residences and would be expected to take a proper proprietorial interest in their property.

The private "homes" and State hospitals will still serve those who do not want anything different. The dower house is not intended as a service like the fire service or even the health service, but is merely a suggestion for a method of procedure whereby the heir can rescue his personal inheritance in a period when it looks very much as if he may lose it. Just now the take-over is being overlaid by a mixed welter of welfare and gracious living, and the principle of the Relay is being forgotten in the middle of its run – which is about as disastrous to the nation as a team doing the same thing in the Olympics.

"A mixed welter"?
Julia Jones

The mixed welter sounds like an event that's not yet been presented to the Olympic committee: a combination of hopscotch, reverse butterfly and the wheelbarrow race, perhaps. Margery's fear in 1964 was that the essential handover from one generation to another was "being overlaid by a mixed welter of welfare and gracious living, and the principle of the Relay is being forgotten". The principle of the Relay is that it is as important for the younger members of a family as it is for the old, that the last months or years of life should be managed as well as the first. Practical arrangements that provide peace, safety, companionship and an essential closeness to whoever is principally taking responsibility will allow the old person to distribute their batons of inheritance and to be "reabsorbed" back into the family "where all that remains of them will survive".

Certainly today we have a mixed welter of practical and financial arrangements. Some people are growing old on generous pensions but many are not. There *is* welfare. More of it and better than in Margery's day – but never sufficient and feeling increasingly precarious and arbitrary. Families who want to support their older members too often find their energies dissipated in confusing battles with assessment panels when they should be working in mutually respectful partnership. The concept of the family has varied since the 1960s and many more types of relationship are publicly accepted.

Family fragmentation has also increased and physical distance between generations is often a major challenge as people work across the world. Nevertheless human affection remains constant and there are hundreds of thousands of family carers doing their personal best to look after the people they love, both in old age and with chronic conditions.[54]

In 1958, when Margery and Joyce accepted responsibility for Em, Maud and Grace, family carers were unrecognised. In January 1963, however, the Rev Mary Webster wrote a letter to *The Times* drawing attention to the plight of unmarried women, like herself, who had given up work to care full time for their parents in old age. Webster described people in her situation as living "under house arrest".[55] In 1965 she founded the National Council for Unmarried Women and their Dependents, the first formal manifestation of what is now the Carers Movement. Unlike the Allinghams' mix of paid and unpaid care, Mary Webster was coping alone. The Allinghams read *The Times* and I cannot help wondering whether the publicity generated by Mary Webster's campaign influenced Margery's counter-insistence on the importance of finding ways in which to manage elder care without putting the rest of one's life on hold.

Although Margery came to feel that *The Relay* was "a bit premature somehow" she was writing in a period of innovation. Richard Carr-Gomm, founder of the Abbeyfield Society, had been developing his vision of "a house in every street" where old people could live safely and companionably within their own communities since 1956. The first recorded use of the

54 Currently 6.8 million according to the most recent estimate from the Carers' Trust. Unpaid carers save the economy annually more than the total annual cost of the NHS.

55 *History of the Carers Movement* Tim Cook (Carers UK 2007)

term "Granny annex" was July 1959 (once again in *The Times*).[56] The adjective "sheltered" was first used in a housing context to describe a hostel in Oxford in 1961 and also appears in Peter Townsend's *The Last Refuge* (1962) as a rare but desirable development to enable old people to remain in the community.[57] Meanwhile Cicely Saunders was working towards establishing the world's first purpose-built hospice.[58] Margery's ideas about the positive importance of family responsibility towards the end of life could also have been heard in this period, but were not.

As soon as *The Relay* was completed in November 1964 she sent it, confidently enough, to her agent, Graham Watson. She had various anxieties about the best way for it to be published without it conflicting with the imminent appearance of *The Mind Readers* but it was not until the spring of 1965 that she began to recognise that there were problems with it appearing at all. "My own bet is that it is a bit premature somehow. Anyway it seems to have taken a weight of my own mind. Am glad to have got it down."[59] She didn't give up on *The Relay* but set it aside. "There is a good deal of interesting stuff in it but it is served up in untidy heaps. Written very fast."[60] She planned to revise it but meanwhile her priority was producing the new, more conventional, detective novel which would have been *Cargo of Eagles*.

56 1959 *Times,* 2 July, 7/4. The perfect answer is for all local authorities to build some "Plus-Granny Annexes"—that is, small independent housing units attached to the side of ordinary family houses.

57 1961 *Oxford Mail,* 16 March, 4/6. The three-storey house [for patients of a mental hospital in the final stages of readjustment to community life]...was opened last month and is known officially as a "sheltered hostel"...

58 St Christopher's Hospice opened in 1967.

59 MA to Graham Watson, letter 6.4.1965.

60 MA to Graham Watson, letter 1.6.1965.

Margery was tired. Although she asserted that *The Mind Readers* was the work of a "Phoenix Marge", by the beginning of 1966 she could no longer hide the fact that she was seriously ill, both mentally and physically. Increasing pain and secret fear spilled into hallucination and paranoia and, in February, she dictated an extraordinary piece of writing, "Queen Beetle", apparently from within a state of near delirium.[61] She was compulsorily admitted to Severalls, the mental hospital in nearby Colchester, and was a patient there for just over a month. This was a significant moment in the abortive history of *The Relay*.

The consultant psychiatrist who had examined Margery at home and had taken the decision that she should be compulsorily detained was Dr Russell Barton. Barton was a passionate advocate for improved conditions in both mental health and geriatric wards and for moving care out of institutions and into the community. He was the author of the seminal 1959 work *Institutional Neurosis*[62] and, since his arrival at Severalls in 1960, had been energetically unlocking wards, organising social events for patients and staff and inviting local people in. Barton was never afraid of controversy and was an essential member of the fledgling campaign Aid for the Elderly in Government Institutions (AEGIS), run by the energetic amateur Barbara Robb.

Robb was an articulate, artistic, reasonably affluent woman living in Hampstead, North London. She was interested in psychology and had become a regular visitor to an elderly seamstress, Amy Gibbs, who had been admitted to Friern

61 *The Adventures of Margery Allingham,* Julia Jones (Golden Duck 2009)

62 Barton's main thesis was that "asylum care generated a neurotic condition in patients over and above their original ill-health." *Institutional Neurosis* (John Wright 1959) It's an understanding that is equally relevant to some of the behaviours associated with dementia.

Hospital in 1963. In the nineteenth century Friern had been the most expensive asylum ever built, an ambitious project and a source of county pride. By the 1960s, however, its fabric had deteriorated and a significant number of patients, particularly those who were old or living with dementia, were there simply because there was nowhere else for them to go. When Barbara Robb visited Amy Gibbs she saw what I remember glimpsing when we visited Granny in her Suffolk ex-workhouse. Lines and lines of beds filled with old people in states of depression, apathy, bewilderment, de-personalisation. "We have all seen wards where the beds are so crowded together that often there is not even room to place lockers between the beds, or where the beds overflow into the corridor of the hospital."[63]

Robb saw more clearly than my parents and I did. She noticed an apparently systematic "stripping" of all the small but essential props that enable old people to continue to function: hearing aids, dentures, money, walking sticks. My parents thought the nurses had "stolen" the nightdresses they had brought for Granny; Barbara Robb believed that the removal of individual clothing and the random reallocation of garments were symptomatic of an underlying callousness, a systemic inhumanity. I went back to my boarding school and wrote a bad poem, Robb began to collect evidence from other concerned relatives and, crucially, from nurses. Soon she was shocked by reports of active brutality as well as the widespread, insidious neglect of the old and the mentally frail, not only in Friern but in other long-stay hospitals throughout the country.

My parents and my uncle muttered to each other about Granny's situation and I remember that she moved from one

63 1965 House of Commons debate on the Mental Health Act, quoted in "Ghettos for Grandparents", *Sans Everything: A Case to Answer* (AEGIS 1967).

ex-workhouse to another, perhaps marginally less grim. I'm not sure because I can't remember ever visiting her again. Barbara Robb began writing letters to the newspapers and collecting supporters and, in November 1965, she founded AEGIS – with Dr Russell Barton as one of its key crusading members. In Severalls, in the early spring of 1966, Margery and Dr Barton developed a cautious patient/doctor friendship as her mental condition stabilised and attempts were made to treat the breast cancer she had been determinedly ignoring since 1955. He visited her regularly in the evenings for absorbing, wide-ranging conversations. *The Relay* became a part of these. Barton read the book, admired it and made some suggestions and clarifications.[64]

Their friendship continued after Margery returned home to D'Arcy House in mid-March. The prognosis was not good and Joyce constructed an *ad hoc* version of the dower house "antechamber" by converting a small wash-house, a few steps from the kitchen door, into a last bedroom. In late June, Margery was readmitted to Severalls for further cancer investigation and there she died. Later that year Dr Barton wrote to Joyce asking her permission for *The Relay* to be published as a contribution to *Sans Everything*, a crusading collection of AEGIS reports on the care of the elderly. He spoke warmly of both Margery and her book. "It was very dear to her heart and I think a most astute analysis of the problems with many excellent and simple solutions."[65]

But Joyce refused. Her reason – the standard one that Margery herself would have understood – was that Pip wouldn't

64 It must have been at this point, or immediately after, that the radical abridgement of *The Relay* from a short book into a long article took place. It was reorganised into headings and became more prescriptive and less discursive.

65 Russell Barton to Joyce Allingham, 1977.

like it and she hadn't the strength to deal with his hostility and objections. Pip and Joyce, separately grief-stricken and mutually incompatible, were working, and to some extent existing, together as they tried to continue the affairs of their company P&M Youngman Carter Ltd. Pip was completing Margery's novel *Cargo of Eagles* but "says it's not a success". Margery had worried about *The Relay* diverting attention from her main job as a detective novelist and Joyce realised that Pip would be more than usually sensitive over the protection of Margery's public image. "It's that damn man Barton spoiling her reputation with those B old people," as she attempted to explain.[66]

Joyce tried to rationalise her refusal and also to compromise but the fact remains this was an unrepeatable missed opportunity. *Sans Everything: A Case to Answer* was published by AEGIS in January 1967. It was the first of what has become a line of highly critical exposés of bad practice within specific geriatric and mental health institutions.[67] Section One, "The Case", included "Cruelty in the Old People's Ward" written by *New Statesman* journalist CH Rolph; "Ghettos for Grandparents" (an AEGIS symposium); then more, harrowing, eyewitness accounts from nurses, social workers, a relative and, finally, Barbara Robb's own diary of her visits to Amy Gibbs. Section Two offered some possible answers, including best practice from the psycho-geriatric unit at Severalls. Inclusion of *The Relay* would have altered *Sans Everything*. Margery's book is so determinedly positive, personal, family-based, human scale.

Barbara Robb had high hopes for her book – as campaigners typically do. Naively, we assume that all we need

66 JA to RB, letter 7.12.1966

67 *Social Policy, Social Welfare and Scandal,* Ian Butler & Mark Drakeford (1988) presents *Sans Everything* as initiating a characteristic pattern of exposure and investigation.

to do is to tell Authority what is wrong, prove our case, get the message to the right people and change will swiftly follow. When Joyce Allingham attempted to soften her refusal by offering permission for *The Relay* to be published by AEGIS at some later date, Robb responded that she hoped by then that the need would have passed.[68] In fact *Sans Everything* sparked anger and denial in official circles. Attempts were made to discredit Robb herself and subsequent investigations into the specific institutions mentioned all concluded that there was no case to answer.

Russell Barton's reforming career continued to inspire and irritate his colleagues. Eventually he fell out with the Board at Severalls and moved to America. His career was influential and distinguished but a codicil to his 2003 obituary for the Royal College of Psychiatrists mentions his personal disappointment at the comparative failure of care in the community for the mentally ill. And care for the old? While no-one could regret the closure of the quasi-Poor Law back-wards which accommodated my grandmother and provoked *Sans Everything*, what would he have thought of the mixed welter of provision that we have now? I met Dr Barton in 1990 when I was researching Margery's biography but missed my opportunity to ask. Still I was only interested in *The Relay* as something Margery had produced, a document that shed light on her life and attitudes, not as an expression of a point of view that has an intrinsic value independent of its author. It was the same mistake that Joyce had made.

It's hard now not to feel a wry kinship with Barbara

68 "If the event must really be postponed for at least three years then, for the old people's sake, we can only most earnestly pray that, by that time, it will no longer be seriously needed as a campaigning instrument" (BR to JA, letter 17.12.1966).

Robb, an outraged member of the liberal middle classes, taking a look at the conditions of old age for the poor and powerless and sweeping off to the Department of Health and Parliamentary Select Committee, in her big hats, saying up with this we will not put. Reformers are earnest, irritating, obsessive. Nicci and I have felt faintly ridiculous as we scurry around the country making statements of the obvious. In 1967 Barbara Robb claimed that housing old people in long wards of sixty to eighty beds, removing their personal possessions, and giving them no occupation or treatment (except for the almost ubiquitous ECT) was not a good model of care. We say that people living with dementia who depend on the love and personal knowledge of their families to function in their daily lives are unlikely to thrive in hospital if this unique source of support and understanding is removed. We hadn't heard of Barbara Robb or Mary Webster when we initiated John's Campaign. Our inspiration came from a different 1960s movement: Mother Care for Children in Hospitals.[69] Again it seems extraordinary that there should ever have needed to be an amateur-fuelled campaign to establish the concept that children in hospital do better when they are not separated from the people they depend upon and love.

Could *The Relay* have changed attitudes towards family involvement and home-scale care at the end of life if it had been published in the 1960s together with *Sans Everything*? Perhaps not. For a campaign to catch hold it needs somehow to be articulating a widespread and current emotion. Mother Care for Children in Hospitals was a response to the experience of family separation during the Second World War

69 Founded in 1961, now Action for Sick Children (www.actionforsickchildren.org.uk).

and a new understanding of attachment theory. Mary Webster's campaign for carer recognition gained energy from the same perceptions of gender inequality that were simultaneously fuelling Women's Liberation. Peter Townsend's *The Last Refuge* and Russell Barton's *Institutional Neurosis* both became standard texts for professionals but their ideas took a decade longer to effect even limited change and longer still to reach the general public – if indeed they have. *The Relay* was never intended to spark a crusade or alter government policy. It's a book for individuals and their families, an odd mix of "God and the drains." Margery's inspiration was urgent but her claims are modest. "The people who know it do not need to be told again and the people who do know it will not learn it by reading."

Speaking only for myself, I don't agree. Of course people learn in many different ways but I have usually learned best from reading. When I was expecting my first child, I read pregnancy, birth and child development books. After DD-day, I read as much as I could bear about the illness and ways to try to live alongside it: *Contented Dementia, Keeper, And Still the Music Plays, Where Memories Go.*[70] It's the Prognosis that makes this so much harder than reading about birth. Dementia is terminal. Whatever you do, it's going to end badly. I should be reading more books about death, I suppose. I know I'm afraid of it and so is my mother.

When I arrived at Deben View recently it was getting towards evening, 5.30pm, that dreaded sundowners time, even when these April evenings are clear and long. My mother had been well looked after by the lassies and the forty-second cousins and was bright enough to say so. She had been walking

70 *Contented Dementia,* Oliver James (Vermilion 2009), *Keeper,* Andrea Gillies (Short Books 2010).

the corridors and fidgeting about, hoping I would come, afraid she might be mistaken. She was tense and tired but holding herself together. Her relief when I arrived was obvious and touching. Once we had made the usual pot of tea and settled on her sofa she talked for a few moments about nothing in particular, then put her hand in mine and closed her eyes with a sigh. It reminded me of a talk given by an Ormiston Trust worker about organising children's visits to their mothers in Holloway. They don't want to do very much, she had said. Most of them just climb onto their mother's lap and fall asleep.

My mother has a nice hand. Her skin is fine and warm and delicate. She's never been much of a one for touching and hugging and neither am I. I remembered afterwards, quite unexpectedly, the moment of relationship which is the finest in our lives – from my perspective. It was when I was in labour, giving birth to my first child and none of it was quite like the books or the ante-natal classes had led me to believe. I was at home, as I'd insisted, and it was that moment of transition before the final stage. I knew I needed to keep calm, keep still and pant. I was on the edge of panic and it was then that Mum slipped her hand in mine. I felt that I was floating. It was an almost out-of-body and beautiful experience, far removed from the dirt and pain. I will be grateful for that moment for ever.

Margery and her mother parted "on good terms" after a difficult lifelong relationship.[71] She wrote *The Relay* after their handover was completed and all her old people were dead. We haven't reached that moment so I don't know how this story ends. Meanwhile *The Relay* has helped me recognise and treasure some unexpected moments of surprised recollection. I think that I may understand Margery's concept of transference

71 Information from Joyce.

and accept that there is gain as well as loss in all of this. I know I will never look at clouds and trees and the sparkle of sunshine on the water in the same way again after the time I have spent watching Mum while she is watching them. The colour of daffodils, the activity of a pigeon outside her window, scraps of song and a breathless absorption in favourite poetry or a children's story... rereading *The Relay* has made me conscious that these are not just incidents; these are gifts.

That's nothing extraordinary. "I always think of dear old so and so when I look at that." You often hear people say such things. There are so many scraps from other people's lives that are woven into our own. John's Campaign has led me a little further into the relationship of family and State as each focuses on the welfare of the oldest members of society and particularly, in this generation, on those whose lives are altered by dementia. The State has made huge advances in its provision of facilities and professions of concern, though there are still the shocking incidences of abuse and neglect that must make Barbara Robb quiver in her grave. There always will be, I fear, as long as there are institutions that are secretive and closed, where power and powerlessness become polarised, unmitigated by the normalcy of family relationships and the observation of caring friends.

Families, too, can go sour if there is no fresh air from outside. The situation of all those invisible, spinster daughters, giving up their lives, careers, financial independence and sexual warmth to their parents was potentially as bad, in its way, as the rows of beds in the workhouse wards. The plight of the full-time carer was blown open by Mary Webster but that's not to say it doesn't still exist. Scottish campaigner Tommy Whitelaw tours the UK reducing audiences to tears with his account of loneliness and desperation as he and his mother struggled to cope with her vascular dementia.[72]

The period of handover naturally makes one think of one's own children – or if there are no children, it may make one wonder who there may be to take responsibility when one is too tired or too muddled to manage alone anymore. Margery had no children. When the end of her life was approaching, aged 62, where I am now, she was deeply reassured by the presence of her younger sister. "Joyce is going to be me," she wrote.

Joyce was also childless – so was their brother Phil. There were no nieces or nephews to do for them what they had done for Maud and Grace. Phil took his life once he realised that his cancer was inoperable. Joyce lived on another thirty years and took particular care to ensure that her own legacies were clear. I know she handed on some batons to me. I was glad to have them and I hope this gave her reassurance. *The Relay* was one, I think. But I have been slow to understand it. I was not prepared for the experience of caring for Mum and however tightly I have clung to Margery's instruction not to "forget to survive", it isn't easy. Again and again, I have discovered the utter dependableness, acceptance and understanding of my partner and my children and their families. I am an ageing woman. There's a significant likelihood that one day they may be asked to care for me. Knowing what I know, how will I bear to accept such emotionally-draining, time-consuming commitment when I become ill or frail?

People who cannot cope alone accept the gift of care because they must. I was astonished by the insight of Naoki Higashida, the autistic teenage author of *The Reason I Jump,* who described his pain at the distress his behaviour caused to

72 http://tommy-on-tour-2011.blogspot.co.uk/

others whilst knowing that he was powerless to modify it.[73] I had stupidly assumed that people with autism were unaware of the feelings of others. I might have thought that about people with dementia but I find that is not so. My mother is uneasy about the time I give her, although she simultaneously depends on it. "But when do you do your work, Jul?" She needs reassurance that I am happy to be with her, that I enjoy our time together, that Francis does not mind. I usually manage to give this – except on the very bad evenings. Reading *The Relay* again, now, has helped convince me that I am indeed benefiting from this unchosen experience. But could I accept such care myself?

Parents learn self-abnegation as a core part of their relationship with their children and it's not easy to change the habits of a lifetime. Nicci has been heard to say that she doesn't want her children to care for her. I wonder whether I would be doing my family a favour if I gave them all a great big hug and headed for the *Dignitas* clinic before I reach my Mayday moment? Imitate the traditional fishermen who didn't try to learn to swim. If their vessel foundered, they filled their boots and went straight down.

John's Campaign is a kitchen-table invention. That's where it began, in family discussion. A few months ago we were once again round a kitchen table talking, this time about our relationships with our parents, the emotional challenge of caring and our undiminished dread of reaching that stage ourselves and becoming dependent on those who are dearest to us. "But what if we *want* to care for you?" asked Anna, one of Nicci's daughters.

It seemed to me unanswerable. We know too much now about the guilt and grief – and even anger – that families feel if

73 *The Reason I Jump,* Naoki Higashida (Sceptre 2014).

.e denied the opportunity to care properly for their loved at the end of life. With an illness such as dementia the of life may be a long time coming, but for many people the nciple remains the same. "The people who know it do not .ed to be told again and the people who do know it will not earn it by reading."

Thank you, Margery Allingham, for writing your experience anyway. And thank you, Mum, for your company on this uncompleted voyage, whether or not we have both been press-ganged on board.

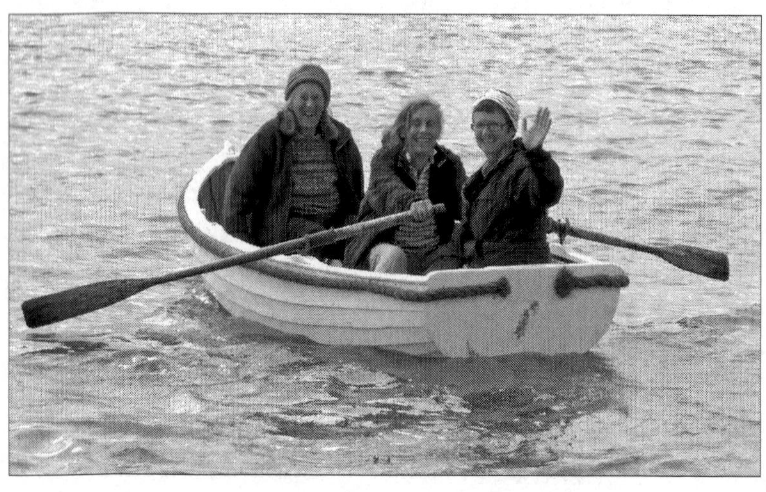

June Jones, Julia Jones, Claudia Myatt, River Deben 2012

Acknowledgements

My greatest debt is to my mother. It's an awkward situation. She knows I am writing this book and approves its title. She won't be able to read it however and if I read it to her there are passages that she would find disconcerting because she has no memory of her bad moments. She remembers her nightmares – that's different unfortunately. She is interested in understanding her condition (when she can cope with hearing about it) and I know she feels proud of the help she has given Nicci and me with John's Campaign (when she can remember what it is). In September 2015 Anglia TV asked us for an interview which I was very reluctant to give yet that turned out to be one of the happiest moments in her recent years. The souvenir photograph has been loved into creases. I hope that, in some way, she will be glad I have been keeping a log of our voyage so far.

About thirty years ago, in my bookseller days, Mum helped me to produce a several volumes of Essex Old People's reminiscence. Both of us felt moved and enlightened by all that we learned from the people who contributed their memories. In this case I have been learning essentially from Margery Allingham and her family but I have also been meeting hospital staff who are challenging themselves to do better for their patients, people with dementia who are determined to live well and families who are caring devotedly for those they love. I wish I could name them all here.

If I were writing reverse acknowledgements I would rant at the low priority given to mental health provision despite political fine words. Currently there is just one specialty doctor single experienced nurse covering later life psychiatry ur whole coastal area. It took from November until ch before Mum and I received the expert help we needed. wever this is a part of the book which should probably main positive. So I will just thank the housing manager, the ocial worker, the dementia specialist, the GP *and* the mental health team who finally enabled us to stabilise a situation which was running beyond my ability to manage.

Throughout this winter my friends at Authors Electric (http://authorselectric.blogspot.co.uk/) have commented with great kindness on a series of blogposts mainly expressing wretchedness and their encouragement was the essential spark for this project. Claudia Myatt's cover design was inspired by Margery's conception of life as a pattern of mixed interconnectedness and separation – which, Margery felt, was particularly well expressed by Paisley. I'm very grateful to Maggie East for allowing me to include her husband Denis's story and to others, such as Sally Magnusson, who have been similarly generous. Thank you to my cousin Gwen Shaw for family memories and to Nigel Cochrane at the Albert Sloman library, Essex University for ready access to the archives. I'm well aware what a boon it is to be able to take the support of the Margery Allingham Society for granted. When I asked Barry Pike, the Chairman, for his blessing on the project he simply said "Do as you think best Julia. I'm sure Joyce would be delighted."

This book owes its particular thanks to Nicci Gerrard, Francis Wheen, Claudia Myatt, Bertie Wheen and Megan Trudell and I need to record my heartfelt personal gratitude to all my family (especially Francis), the Deben View "lassies" and the "forty-second cousins". Don't stop now.